HEALTH IN ALL POLICIES: REPORT ON PERSPECTIVES AND INTERSECTORAL ACTIONS IN THE SOUTH-EAST ASIA REGION

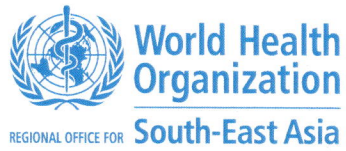

WHO Library Cataloguing-in-Publication data

World Health Organization, Regional Office for South-East Asia.

Health in all policies: report on perspectives and intersectoral actions in the South-East Asia Region.

1. Health Policy – trends - economics 2. Primary Health Care 3. Health Systems Agencies 4. Health Promotion 5. Bhutan 6. India 7. Nepal 8. Sri Lanka 9. Thailand 10. Timor-Leste

ISBN 978-92-9022-448-8   (NLM classification: WA 525)

© **World Health Organization 2013**

All rights reserved.

Requests for publications, or for permission to reproduce or translate WHO publications – whether for sale or for noncommercial distribution – can be obtained from Bookshop, World Health Organization, Regional Office for South-East Asia, Indraprastha Estate, Mahatma Gandhi Marg, New Delhi 110 002, India (fax: +91 11 23370197; e-mail: bookshop@searo.who.int).

The designations employed and the presentation of the material in this publication do not imply the expression of any opinion whatsoever on the part of the World Health Organization concerning the legal status of any country, territory, city or area or of its authorities, or concerning the delimitation of its frontiers or boundaries. Dotted lines on maps represent approximate border lines for which there may not yet be full agreement.

The mention of specific companies or of certain manufacturers' products does not imply that they are endorsed or recommended by the World Health Organization in preference to others of a similar nature that are not mentioned. Errors and omissions excepted, the names of proprietary products are distinguished by initial capital letters.

All reasonable precautions have been taken by the World Health Organization to verify the information contained in this publication. However, the published material is being distributed without warranty of any kind, either expressed or implied. The responsibility for the interpretation and use of the material lies with the reader. In no event shall the World Health Organization be liable for damages arising from its use.

This publication does not necessarily represent the decisions or policies of the World Health Organization.

Design and layout: L'IV Com Sàrl, Villars-sous-Yens, Switzerland

Printed in India

CONTENT

Acknowledgments ii

Abbreviations iii

Introduction 1

1. Historical development of health in all policies in the South-East Asia Region 2
   1.1. Preliminary evidence of a whole-of-government approach 3
   1.2. Preliminary evidence of intersectoral action as part of primary health care and
        Universal Health Coverage 4
   1.3. WHO Regional Office for South-East Asia contributions 6

2. Current perspectives on intersectoral action experiences and health in all policies 7

3. Implementation Experiences: intersectoral/multisectoral actions for health and addressing
   the social determinants of health 10
   3.1. Primary Health Care and Universal Health Coverage 10
   3.2. Prevention and control of the global burden of disease 12
   3.3. Risk factors 12
   3.4. Health promotion and healthy public policies 16
   3.5. Intersectoral actions addressing determinants of health 18

4. Fostering factors, building blocks and drivers for implementation of HiAP 20
   4.1. Creating opportunities 20
   4.2. Legislative framework 21
   4.3. Institutional intersectoral mechanisms 22
   4.4. Joint, innovative financial mechanism 22
   4.5. Capacity & human resources 22

5. Impacts and Lesson Learns 24
   5.1. Political will and process 24
   5.2. Health promotion, health equity and Primary Health Care 24
   5.3. Economic and social change 25
   5.4. Capacity building 26

6. South-East Asia Regional Framework for Health in All Policies 27

7. Way forward 30

Annex 1: Summary of case studies 32
Annex 2: South-East Asia Region Statement on Health in All Policies 41

Bibliography 43

Tables and figures

Table 1. Primary Health care and Universal Health Coverage in the South-East Asia Region
and implications for intersectoral action 11
Figure 1. Regional framework on Health in All Policies 29

ACKNOWLEDGEMENTS

This document was prepared with the support of the Rockefeller Foundation (grant no. 2012 THS 317) as part of the Rockefeller Transforming Health Systems Initiative, *Supporting the Development of Regional Positions on Health in All Policies and Identifying Lessons and Opportunities for Implementation* (*Supporting Regional Positions on Health in All Policies*, for short). The grant, received by the Department of Ethics and Social Determinants of Health of the World Health Organization (WHO), aimed to support evidence-informed decisions in three WHO regions related to how governments can enhance intersectoral approaches to improve health and health equity through implementing a Health in All Policies approach: Africa (AFR), South-East Asia (SEAR) and the Western Pacific (WPR). The products produced using this grant provided support to WHO offices and Ministries of Health to conduct and to document analyses of intersectoral action and Health in All Policies, and to hold intercountry policy discussions relevant to implementing a Health in All Policies approach. It supported several policy dialogues leading up to and during the WHO 8th Global Conference on Health Promotion in Helsinki in 2013.

The project team, coordinated by Ms Nicole Valentine (principal investigator) of the Department of Ethics and Social Determinants of Health (ESD), included, for WHO headquarters, Mr Tomas Allen (librarian), Xenia de Graaf (intern) and Dr Orielle Solar; for the regions: Dr Davison Munadowafa (WHO), who coordinated the project work for WHO in the African Region, and Dr Peter Phori (WHO), Dr Suvajee Good (WHO), who coordinated the project work in South-East Asia Region, Dr Shilpa Modi Pandav, Professor KR Nayar, Ms Anjana Bhushan (WHO), who coordinated the project work for WHO in the Western Pacific Region, and Ms Britta Baer (WHO), Professor Sharon Friel, Mr Patrick Harris and Ms Sarah Simpson. Technical inputs to the project and contributions from other WHO staff in disseminating this work are gratefully acknowledged. Dr Sofia Leticia Morales, of the Pan American Health Organization, offered valuable advice in the set-up of the project. Also, particular thanks go to the following WHO staff for their advice and support in dissemination: for headquarters, Dr KC Tang (coordinator, Health Promotion) and Dr Timo Ståhl (Health Promotion), Dr Rüdiger Krech (Director, ESD) and Eugenio Villar (coordinator, Social Determinants of Health), and in the Western Pacific Region, Dr Katrin Engelhardt and Dr Temo Waqanivalu.

This principal writer of this report was Dr Suvajee Good, Programme Coordinator (Health Promotion) and Social Determinants of Health Focal Point (WHO SEAR). The writing of the report draws upon two commissioned reports reviewing intersectoral action in the region. The writers of the other reports were Dr KR Nayar (India) and Dr Shilpa Modi Pandav (Timor-Leste). It also uses information and inputs from two regional meetings, case studies and interviews. The cases upon which this report is also based were written by Mr Sonam Rinchen, Bhutan; Mr Shiva Raj Adhikari, Institute of Nepal Environment and Health System Development, Nepal; Ms Anushree Mishra India; Professor Dr Rajitha Wickremasinghe, University of Kelaniya, Sri Lanka; Dr Tipicha Posayanonda, Dr Nattaya Thaennin, Dr Orapan Srisookwantana, IHPP-MOPH, Thailand; and by Dr Shilpa Modi Pandav, Timor-Leste.

The assistance of WHO headquarters through the WHO Kobe Centre is also acknowledged with thanks. The WHO Kobe Centre provided financial support for the development of two of the country case studies discussed in this report.

The work of the various country offices is also acknowledged with gratitude. This includes technical, administrative and financial support from the WHO Country Office for Bhutan; the WHO Country Office for India; the WHO Country Office for Nepal; the WHO Country Office for Sri Lanka; the WHO Country Office for Thailand; and the WHO Country Office for Timor-Leste.

ABBREVIATIONS

AIDS	Acquired Immunodeficiency Syndrome
CSDH	The Commission on Social Determinants of Health
FCTC	WHO Framework Convention on Tobacco Control
GNH	Gross National Happiness
GNHC	Gross National Happiness Commission
HEA	Health equity audits /assessment
HIA	Health impact assessment
HiAP	Health in All Policies
HIV	Human Immunodeficiency Virus
HLA	Health lens analysis,
HSRO	National Health System Reform Office
ISA	Intersectoral action
MDG	Millennium Development Goals
NCD	Noncommunicable diseases
NGO	Non-governmental organizations
NHA	National Health Assembly
PHC	Primary Health Care
SDH	Social determinants of health
SEARO	WHO Regional Office for South-East Asia
UHC	Universal Health Coverage
UNDAF/UNPAF	United Nations Development/Partnership Frameworks
WHA	World Health Assembly
WHO	World Health Organization

INTRODUCTION

This report presents an analysis of the state of intersectoral action and Health in All Policies in the South-East Asia Region, with a view to building the case for increased reinforcement of the steps being taken by governments to implement Health in All Policies, as called for in the Helsinki Statement on Health in All Policies (2013).

The analyses conducted for the report included literature reviews, key informant interviews, in-depth case studies and country consultations. The country consultations included two regional meetings and a side meeting in Finland.

The report analyses the strengths and weaknesses of intersectoral work in the regional context, and how it can be strengthened towards applying a Health in All Policies approach across public policies.

1. HISTORICAL DEVELOPMENT OF HEALTH IN ALL POLICIES IN THE SOUTHEAST ASIA REGION

Countries in the WHO South-East Asian Region have a long history and much experience of intersectoral/multisectoral actions[1] for disease control and public health interventions spanning back to the 1970s. As a region, South-East Asia comprises 11 Member States, each at different levels of development with disparities across and within countries. Countries in South East Asia are diverse in terms of population size, political structure, economic development, and social and cultural conditions. Bhutan, Democratic People's Republic of Korea, Myanmar, Nepal, and Timor-Leste are categorized as least developed countries, while others such as Bangladesh, India, Indonesia, Maldives and Thailand are classified as countries with emerging economies. Thus, the two groups have varying degrees of dependence on external or donor economic support. Geographically, they differ due to their unique environments and natural resources which make them rich yet they are also vulnerable because of natural disasters. Overall, the importance of different determinants of health vary, and quality of life also differs across these countries.

Government responses to population health requirements in countries are seen to be shaped by their governance structures, human capacities, and resources. Health is seen as a positive concept that can also draw attention to other sectors outside health.

There is clear evidence, from the review of peer literature over the past decades, of intersectoral interventions established to address maternal and child health, nutrition programmes, controlling communicable diseases such as HIV/AIDS, dengue fever, tuberculosis and the prevention of communicable diseases through water and sanitation programmes in the region.

Over the past decades, intersectoral collaboration between Ministries of Health and Education is one of the success stories, which demonstrates how education, particularly female education at secondary level, has reduced maternal and child mortality in a number of countries in the Region. Given how female education is strongly correlated with development, "Health for All" and "Education for All" approaches were synchronized in a way that made tackling determinants of health and raising national development in the Region possible. Yet it is acknowledged, as elsewhere, that many challenges still remain to improve gender equity.

More recently, the Bangkok Charter on Health Promotion (2005) has been a benchmark for health promotion activities in South-East Asia and called for participation of all stakeholders, to take action on healthy public policies. Healthy settings, namely schools, cities, communities and hospitals began to coordinate and collaborate, leading to some institutionalization of structures and processes between health and other sectors. There is evidence that similar intersectoral processes exist in India, Indonesia, Sri Lanka, and Thailand. In the South-East Asia Region, a series of consultations on social determinants of health were conducted in 2007 and 2009 to discuss

---

1 While intersectoral action is a well-established term in public health, the term "multisectoral action" has also gained frequency of usage in health policy forums. For the purposes of the Global Conference on Health Promotion, multisectoral and intersectoral action terms were used as synonyms. However, multisectoral action can have the interesting connation of public service agencies acting *simultaneously*.

how to address health inequities and determinants of health. In February 2009, the WHO Regional Consultation on Social Determinants of Health assessed actions taken by Member States to reduce the equity gap. These consultations identified a number of examples ranging from a contributory social security system for self-employed women in India, micro-credit for the poorest in Bangladesh, and provision of universal health care in Thailand. The consultation resulted in the "Colombo Call for Action" which urged countries to mainstream "health equity in all policies", empower individuals and communities, and advocate for good governance and corporate social responsibility. Subsequently, Sri Lanka launched the so-called "Lighthouse Project" to address socio-economic and cultural factors in relation to all priority areas of determinants of health, which involved several studies and operational research. A series of studies and analyses on social disparities and equity were also conducted in the Region.

Despite a long historical experience with intersectoral action, only a few countries have explicitly adopted healthy public policies, Health in All Policies or a whole-of-government approach to address population health and the underlying social determinants in the Region. From the regional literature review and research conducted in 2012–2013, Thailand is the only country in the South-East Asia Region that has applied a legislative framework to ensure the health of its population. The framework uses health impact assessment to ensure healthy public policies are promoted in the country. Bhutan, Sri Lanka, and Timor-Leste have used different whole-of-government approaches to support intersectoral action to improve the health and well-being of their people.

However, there has been limited knowledge on how the approach has been implemented and therefore no systematic report on progress toward achieving healthy public policies or Health in All Policies in these countries.

1.1 Preliminary evidence of a whole-of-government approach

Historically, public health in South-East Asia has been an important indicator of national development. Improving quality of life through public health and social services has always been the mission of the governments, especially between the 1960s and 1980s. The first country example to illustrate this was Sri Lanka. Two decades after the independence of Sri Lanka between 1950 and 1975, Sri Lanka underwent a rapid health transition that was characterized by prolonged life and reduced mortality.[2] The average life expectancy of the population increased from 55.6 years to 67.1 years at birth, infant mortality dropped from 5.6 to 1.0 per 1000 live births, and fertility declined from 5.0 to 3.4 births per woman between 1963 and 1974 (Gunatilleke 1984). The Government of Sri Lanka adopted a holistic social welfare approach supported by a broad set of social policies to address health, education, food security, and meet the basic needs of the population. There was a high level of political commitment for social welfare programmes which led to signs of improvement. The Cabinet was the forum in which inter-ministerial coordination took place and the system ensured that all important policy decisions were taken collectively. Cooperation between ministries was sought between and among sectors, on an ad hoc basis, to deliver the services. The main intersectoral mechanism operating in the 1980s was the District Coordinating Committee which had representatives from all the government departments. The Committee was responsible for solving and responding to needs of people within a locality.

In 2007, the Thailand National Health Act was promulgated and widely considered to be a landmark of health leadership in how to institutionalize multisectoral action. It took over a decade to deliver. The concept of "healthy public policy development" had been raised in Thailand in the mid-1980s, however active participation from communities came only after the Constitution of the Kingdom of Thailand in 1997. Under the Constitution, the National Health System Reform Committee and the National Health System Reform Office were established in 2000. The National Health System

---

2 Shilpa Modi Pandav (2012) *Draft Documentation on Implementation of Health in All Policies in the South-East Asia Region*, commissioned by WHO-SEARO, September 2012

Reform Committee consisted of health personnel, academics, civil society groups, multistakeholders from different sectors and partners engaged in health reform activities, which included the drafting of the National Health Act. The process of drafting the Act involved active multi-stakeholder participation with over 500 brainstorming sessions with more than 400 000 participants.[3] The Act served as an effective tool to set guidance on the National Health Development in which all parties in society should be involved throughout the participatory process. The Act has also been an instrument for a paradigm shift in the perspective of health, which became operationalized in a broader sense, to encompass physical health, mental health, social and spiritual health understanding of an interrelated holistic view of the individual, family, community, and broader society. Chuengsatiansup (2008) analysed that *"the most important aspect of mobilization of civil society in healthy systems reform was the creation of the civic deliberation process,"* which was reflected in a series of health assemblies in Thailand. The National Health Assembly (NHA) is an important mechanism using an intersectoral approach for development of participatory healthy public policies in Thailand starting in 2008.

Thailand is also the only country in the WHO South-East Region to adopt health impact assessment (HIA) at the highest level of decision-making through legislation, namely the Constitution of the Kingdom of Thailand 2007 and the National Health Act 2007. Section 67 of the Constitution clearly states that health assessment needs to be conducted on *"any project or activity which may seriously affect a community's environmental quality, its natural resources, or its people's health…"* The National Health Act 2007 also endorses that *"an individual or group of people has the right to request an assessment and to participate in the assessment of the health impact resulting from a public policy. …"* Thus, health impact assessment in Thailand became a participatory process in which community awareness of health and well-being is at the centre of the development. After public review, the HIA report and public comments are sent to an environmental impact assessment and health impact assessment technical expert for approval and decision-making in the Cabinet. HIA in Thailand has to be implemented before, during and after development projects. Local administrations such as municipalities, subdistrict administrative organizations, and provincial administration can undertake HIA for a wide range of development policies, projects or activities to ensure there is no health impact associated with local developments.

Similarly, Bhutan's unique philosophy "Gross National Happiness" (GNH) has become the key value of all development policies and plans in Bhutan. The GNH development model has four pillars, including equitable and balanced socioeconomic development, conservation of the natural environment, preservation of culture, and promotion of good governance. A set of nine domains: health, education, living standards, ecology, culture, community, psychological well-being, and time are used to measure the GNH of the country. The Gross National Happiness Commission (GNHC) is the apex body responsible for coordinating and formulating all policies, plans and programmes in the country. It must ensure that all development programmes have no or minimal negative impact on the nine domains of happiness and that they contribute to the country's Gross National Happiness. The GNHC developed the GNH policy screening tool which is used to assess all policies in all sectors and has been in operation since 2010.

1.2 Preliminary evidence of intersectoral action as part of primary health care and Universal Health Coverage

Evidence from past experience in the South-East Asian Region shows that much of the work with other sectors or of whole-of-government approaches has been focused around improving primary health care, in particular for maternal and child health and controlling pandemic diseases, such as HIV/AIDS. The Primary Health Care (PHC) approach has placed national health development within the overall social and economic development since 1978, following the Alma Alta Declaration. The PHC approach was used in the region to address

---

[3] Tipicha Posayanonda, Nattaya Thaennin, Orapan Srisookwatana (2012) *Thailand's National Health Assembly: Intersectoral Action for Health*. Commissioned by WHO-SEARO. Funded by WHO-Kobe Centre, December 2012.

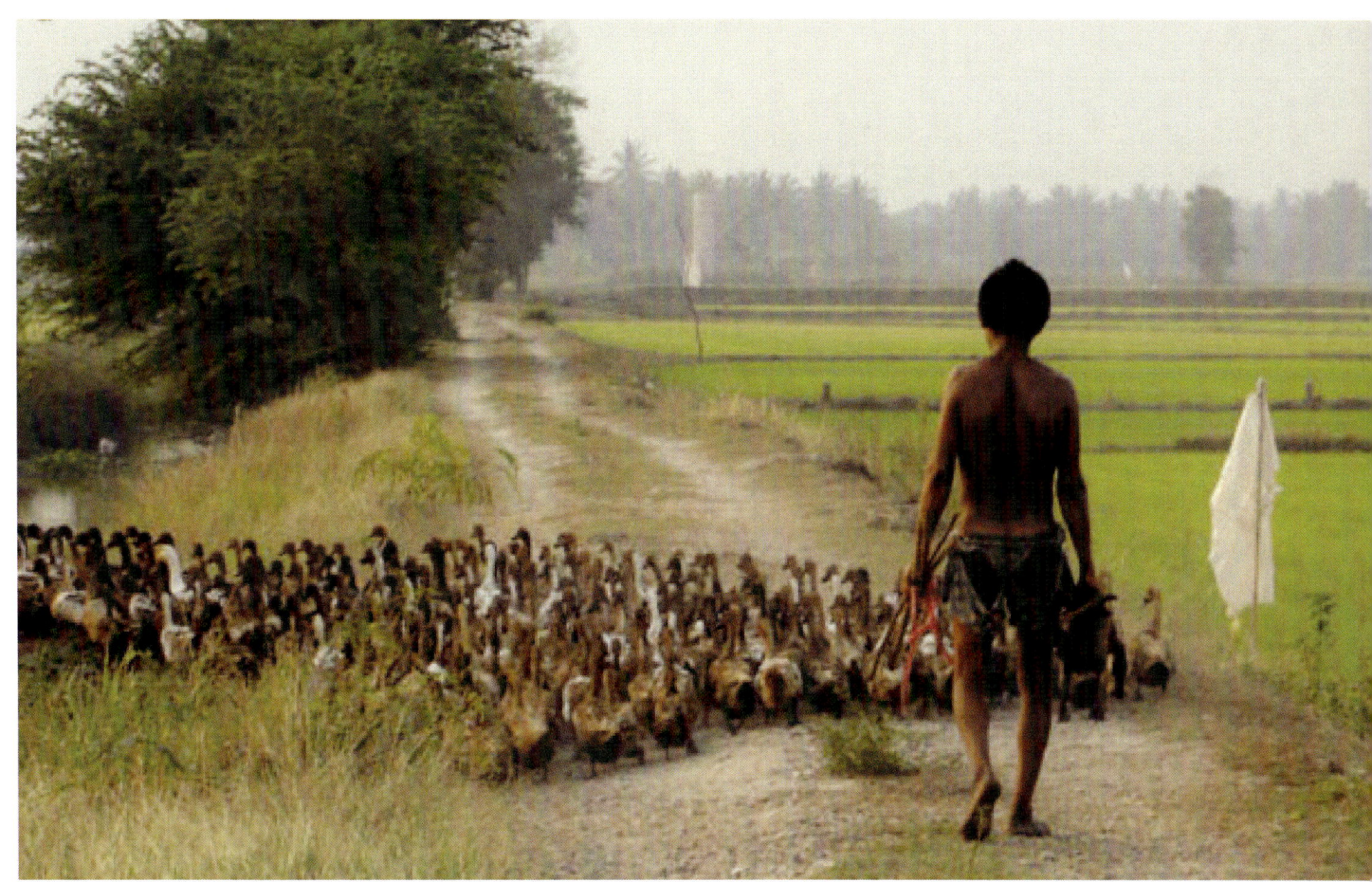

Avian influenza in Thailand. ©WHO/SEARO/Aphaluck Bhatiasevi

health inequity with the appropriate technology, community participation, intersectoral collaboration, and universal coverage approach. It dealt with various health risks, the factors and social determinants affecting health. The PHC approach was used to collaborate with various other sectors, particularly education, water and sanitation, nutrition, agriculture, and local administration.

All WHO South-East Asia Region Member States affirmed their commitment to revitalizing PHC as an effective approach to strengthen systems in 2008[4]. For example, Bhutan has developed strategies to reach the unreached through decentralization of planning and management systems to expand health and other services across countries. The National Rural Health Mission of India was launched in 2005 to provide accessible, affordable, and accountable quality health services inclusive of the poorest households in the remotest rural regions. The Government of Nepal decentralized health systems management, increasing public-private partnerships in the delivery of primary health services across countries. Sri Lanka made remarkable efforts to scale up accessibility and coverage of primary health care to tackle several health problems. The Ministry of Health in Sri Lanka took the lead in planning and sponsoring national behavioural change communication programmes, setting up healthy lifestyle activities among target populations. Thailand strengthened primary health care with a strategic road map increasing competencies of health personnel, improving primary health facilities, establishing referral coordinating centres, and integrating community-based preventive and health promotion with traditional medicine in primary health centres around the country.

Despite the fact that these improvements in primary health care were led by the health sector in the countries, there was evidence that getting other sectors on board required substantial engagement and convincing of intersectoral collaboration with various other sectors beyond health actors.

---

[4] WHO held a Regional Conference on Revitalizing Primary Health Care in Jakarta, Indonesia, in August 2008 (see WHO (2009).

1.3 WHO Regional Office for South-East Asia contributions

In August 2011, a Regional Consultation on Intersectoral Actions Addressing Social Determinants of Health was held in WHO Regional Office for South-East Asia, India. This meeting aimed to support Member States to document the strategies and examples of action they have taken to address the social determinants of health through intersectoral actions. Examples included action to prevent and control communicable and noncommunicable diseases, addressing maternal and child health, and health systems in the region. The meeting enabled Member States to assess the level of implementation of Health in All Policies and action to address the determinants of health in their countries, according to WHA62.14. The consultation resulted in reconfirming Member States' commitment to progress the Health in All Policies approach and to mainstream action on the social determinants of health across sectors.

Yet in spite of these commitments by the health sector, a number of lessons were learned from more recent literature reviews that showed the ineffectiveness of national bodies and mechanisms when they are not well coordinated or have sufficient understanding of, or the mindset for, improving population health. Where health was not the main concern of other sectors, which had their own priorities and issues to deal with, coordination remained a challenge, particularly when the policies of other sectors have direct effects on social determinants of health, such as education, safe and quality housing, sanitation and infrastructure, employment and social insurance. Further, advocacy for health in other sectors will continue to be important to achieve the global commitment. Recommendations from the Regional Consultation on Intersectoral Actions Addressing Social Determinants of Health held in WHO Regional Office for South-East Asia in August 2011 called upon WHO to provide technical support to build the capacity of Member States to assess health impacts and health equity and to move towards Health in All Policies.

Moreover, the UN Summit on Noncommunicable Diseases (NCD) in 2011 unprecedentedly recognized the emergence of four major disease groups, namely cardiovascular diseases, cancer, diabetes, and chronic respiratory diseases as a global problem. Causes of these diseases are preventable, particularly through primary and secondary intervention outside the health sector. The Global Plan of Action for the Prevention and Control of Noncommunicable Diseases is currently being drafted and includes strategies to prevent noncommunicable diseases through applying a Health in All Policies approach. Member States are well aware of the need to address health issues in collaboration with other sectors, and the call for Health in All Policies is crucial.

A Meeting of Experts on Health in All Policies in December 2012, held in Thailand, was an important occasion, as it provided the opportunity to document the implementation of HiAP, including lessons learned, and the drafting of a framework for regional action towards Health in All Policies within the context of the South-East Asia Region. Between June 2012 and April 2013, a series of country case studies, which aimed to document regional policy-level action with a focus on determinants of health using intersectoral approaches, identified a number of emerging and potential practices on how to apply Health in All Policies in the Region. These emerging practices particularly drew on the historical experiences of primary health care, prevention and control of pandemic diseases, movement towards health systems reform, promotion of Universal Health Coverage, and the International Health Regulations (2005). The framework for Health in All Policies for South-East Asia was developed in the Regional Consultation on Health in All Policies in South-East Asia in April 2013, held in Sri Lanka. The Framework and statement was launched in the 8th Global Conference on Health Promotion in June 2013, in Helsinki, Finland. The Regional Framework adapts and summarizes emerging guidance on strategic directions that the Member States could adopt for implementation plans of action appropriate for country priorities in the coming years.

2.
CURRENT PERSPECTIVES ON INTERSECTORAL ACTION EXPERIENCES AND HEALTH IN ALL POLICIES

Although there is rich historical evidence of intersectoral actions in the Region, there is no explicit recognition of HiAP in policy documents, except in Thailand. In a recent review from the European Observatory on Health Systems and Policies and through in-depth interviews, high ranking officials, senior health officials and practitioners in the region expressed their different perspectives on the Health in All Policies approach, which was explained to them in terms of the key elements that were discussed as part of what became the definition used at the Helsinki meeting: "an approach to public policies across sectors that systematically takes into account the health implications of decisions, seeks synergies, and avoids harmful health impacts, in order to improve population health and health equity."

A senior official from India stressed that intersectoral actions which produced desirable results should be recognized as a joint effort, contributed to by all sectors involved not only during the implementation but also in planning and designing the process. In Sri Lanka, the whole-of-government and determinants focus of the approach was reflected in the document under the WHO Commission on Social Determinants of Health *"underlines a growing consensus about the importance of key determinants of health such as income, education, social support networks, employment and working conditions, which are the purview of many different sectors; the need to reduce persistent health status disparities; our increasing understanding of the conditions which enable effective intersectoral action; and a positive climate for action."* [1]

A senior health official from Myanmar considers *"cooperation between health sector and other sectors as the basis of HiAP. This is much more doable in the country's context as usually the health sector has to start and lead the cooperation between different relevant sectors inside and outside the domain of public health regarding aspects of health. Each and other sectors that could influence the determinants of health would collaborate if health could take the lead to dialogue for further process to improve, protect or promote health."* [2]

The Royal Government of Bhutan indicated they had always accorded health a high priority. The Bhutanese policy-makers and planners believe that *"the HiAP approach can be one of the potential tools that may help bridge the gaps of health inequities in the country. The health sector alone cannot address the issue on health inequity because most of the determinants lie in the sectors outside health, such as environment, education, agriculture, trade, governance, etc. Health inequity is indeed the broader concern of the society or the nation at large that needs attention of all pertinent stakeholders."* [3] However some officials thought that simply having HiAP in place may not automatically guarantee a change in priority-setting for health in the current

---
1 Perera MALR (2006). *Intersectoral action for health in Sri Lanka, paper prepared for the WHO Commission on Social Determinants of Health, Health Systems Knowledge Network.*
2 Questionnaire response from Ministry of Health, Myanmar, March 2013.
3 Rinchen, S (2013) Case Study on *"Implementation of Tobacco Control Policy in Bhutan: A Vital Platform for Intersectoral Actions"*, commissioned by WHO-SEARO, March 2013.

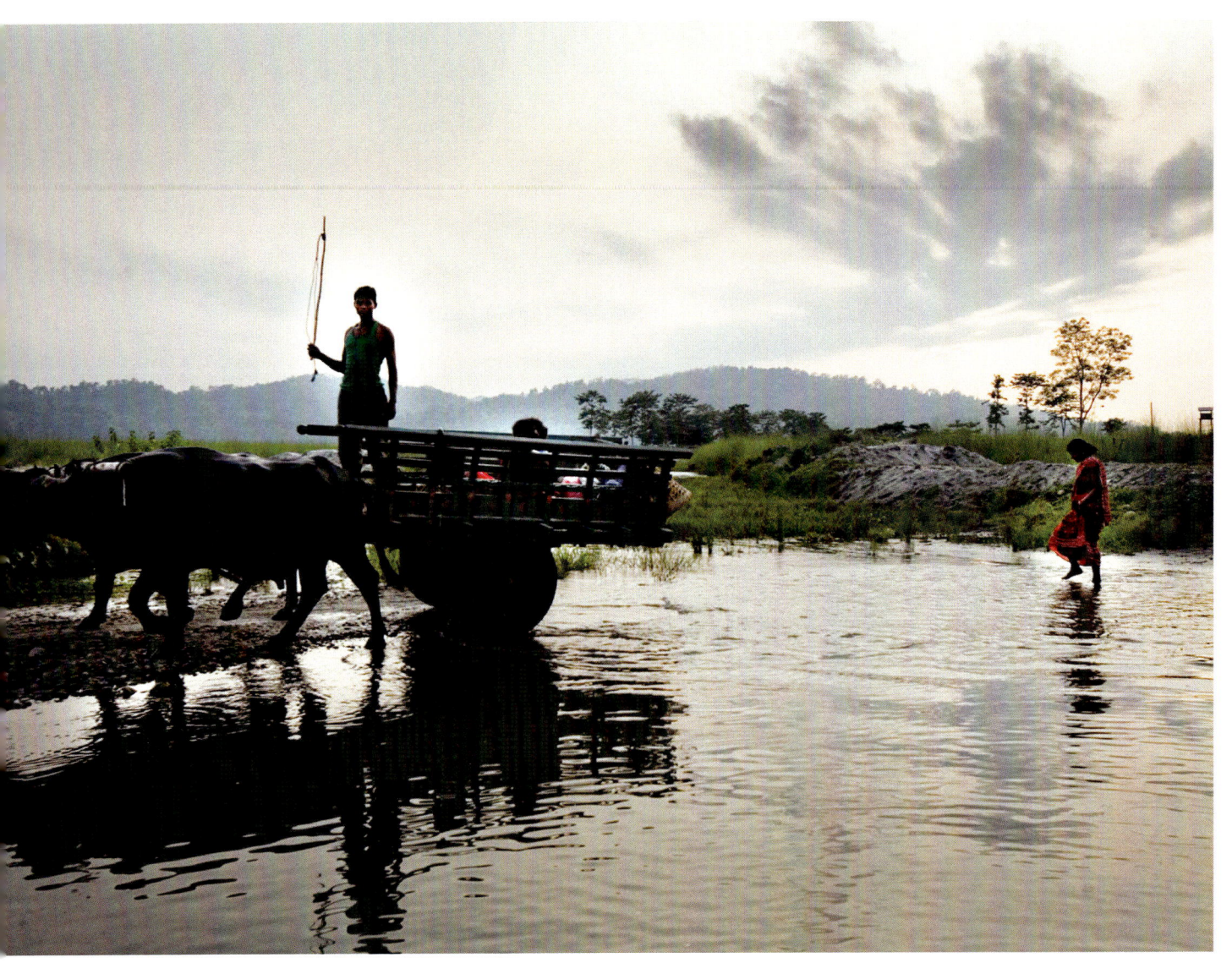

A man rides his ox cart through a river, with his wife walking behind in Nepal. ©Kate Holt/IRIN

government systems. There could be some resistance to change from other sectors, which are unwilling to accept new initiatives. Thus, many viewed that *"HiAP may sustain and work better if it is built on the existing mechanisms, such as (the existing) multisectoral approach for policy implementation, and the GNH's Policy Screening Tool."*[4].

In the case of Thailand, the principles of a people-centred approach and "sufficient economy" were adopted in many national policies. "Sufficient economy" became a shared vision across sectors. Political will and administrative and technocratic competence were contributing factors to the holistic approach to health and its national outcome. Interventions from the non-health sector, such as poverty eradication, improving the literacy rate, gender equality, social inclusion, public infrastructure, reducing gaps between rural and urban communities, and many programmes significantly, although indirectly, influenced the health outcomes. Most of the interventions addressing determinants of health were achieved by non-health sectors, although in some parts were realized together with the health sector. There is a clear understanding and recognition of intersectoral actions and Health in All Policies in Thailand (Nayar, 2013)[5].

A senior official in Thailand accepted WHO's definition on Health in All Policies and expressed that *"HiAP is a strategy that allows the formulation of public policies in sectors other than*

---

4 Rinchen, S (2013). Case Study on *"Implementation of Tobacco Control Policy in Bhutan: A Vital Platform for Intersectoral Actions"*, commissioned by WHO Office for South-East Asia, March 2013, and being prepared for publication.

5 Nayar KR (2013) Working paper on *"Health in All Policies Approach and Intersectoral Actions in South-East Asia Region"*, commissioned by WHO-SEARO, March 2013.

health. If the policies are used correctly, it will have a positive influence on the determinants of health." [6] Experiences from Thailand indicate that major factors stimulating collaboration between different sectors are the presence of non-hierarchical administrative structures, less dependency on external resources, a sense of ownership, political context of the time, and perceived mutual benefits.

Intersectoral actions in Sri Lanka are highly recognized, particularly with the leading role of the Ministry of Health and health-related ministries. Donor assistance for implementing welfare projects and public programmes, such as water supply, sanitation, and housing has contributed to health outcomes. There are many positive trends in health status that have been associated with improvements of welfare measures, free public sector health and social services and free education (Fernando, 2001). As part of the strategy for intersectoral actions and coordination at all levels, the Government of Sri Lanka established the National Health Development Network, with the National Health Council as the apex body, chaired by the Prime Minister. Intersectoral committees have been set up to address major issues in communicable and non-communicable disease controls, prevention of injuries, school health, nutrition, and other programmes. The committees meet on a regular basis to ensure intersectoral collaboration and policy are harmonized. In this sense, the Health in All Policies approach is reflected in intersectoral work for health that is underway in Sri Lanka.

Nongovernmental organizations (NGOs) in Nepal reflected that Health in All Policies could be challenged by "bringing together various actors under one umbrella, given the multitude of NGOs operating with conflicting interests". Conflict of interests not only among the NGOs but also of government agencies regarding the different priority could be a barrier. However, academics and researchers could play important roles in Nepal, if they were to take serious steps to understand policy gaps, and bring together multistakeholders to look at the broader agenda. An activist from the media in Nepal commented that *"public health is generally an 'apolitical' issue and focused on behavioural modification"*. Within the interest groups, some intersectoral collaboration took place in health programmes. However, a certain difficulty reflected during an interview, was the lack of integrated movement to increase the profile of public health issues and the interest of other sectors, which could have been relevant to education, gender, human rights, and child labour.

The response from an Indian health activist and researcher showed that there was a need to prioritize social determinants of health within the health sector itself. *"A prioritization of social determinants of health within the health sector will give other sectors a fair chance to participate in the health planning and in implementation"*, particularly with housing development, education, and food security. However, another professional with grass-roots experience says that *"there is a lack of common understanding for needs, problems, methods and solutions. Unless, there is an open-door policy on sharing funds at local level, intersectoral actions cannot be initiated at local level"* [7].

---

6 Questionnaire response from Ministry of Public Health, Thailand, March 2013.

7 These quotations are extracted from a report commissioned by WHO (see Nayar (2013)

3. IMPLEMENTATION EXPERIENCES: INTERSECTORAL/MULTISECTORAL ACTIONS FOR HEALTH AND ADDRESSING THE SOCIAL DETERMINANTS OF HEALTH

One starting point for applying a Health in All Policies Approach focuses directly on the social determinants of health and work to improve public policies and priorities across government. This includes in education, agriculture, employment policies, which ultimately strengthen the social determinants of health and improve long-term health outcomes. The examples of the HiAP approach in Bhutan and Thailand are aligned closely to this first approach, placing a strong emphasis on improving the overall development within the country by addressing the social determinants of health, and thus contributing to health and other outcomes. The second starting point adopts a focus on a specific health issue and/or goal, which requires intersectoral collaboration and partnership to be achieved. Improvements to the social determinants of health are important, but secondary to achieving positive improvements in specific health issues and/or goals. Prevention of communicable and noncommunicable disease controls, interventions and revitalization of primary health care are examples of the second group.

3.1 Primary health care and Universal Health Coverage

The primary health care (PHC) agenda has been the main mover for actions to address determinants in other policy sectors for more than three decades. Primary health care has advocated and implemented the following approaches: a) universal coverage, b) intersectoral collaboration, c) community participation, and d) appropriate technology.

In Bangladesh, for example, development of the national health system has given high priority to ensuring universal accessibility to, and equity in, health care. In India, the National Rural Health Mission and current health mission have highly emphasized Universal Health Coverage, aiming to provide accessible, affordable, and accountable quality of care.

In Indonesia, Alert Village programme, (Desa Siaga) is an important platform for multisectoral actions for the population's health, and for bringing out a number of decrees and legislation to ensure a wide range of public health issues are considered.

Bhutan has extended primary health care units to remote areas, ensuring access to health services, whereby health professionals and workers coordinate with other sectors to deliver services.

Systematic intersectoral and multisectoral approaches to public health in Sri Lanka and Thailand have been implemented with strong collaboration across relevant departments and agencies, and with community participation.

In Nepal, primary intervention for malnutrition happened with a multisectoral plan and programme featuring intersectoral actions. The National Planning Commission was at the apex of coordinating mechanisms, in which key ministries, such as the Ministry of Health and Population,

Table 1. Primary Health care and Universal Health Coverage in the South-East Asia Region and implications for intersectoral action

Country	Initiatives	Examples of intersectoral action or Health in All Policies implications
Bangladesh	National health systems development has given high priority to ensuring universal accessibility to and equity in health care, with particular attention to the rural population.	Coordination and planning with district governments – whole-of-government approach at the local level
Bhutan	Bhutan has evolved strategies to reach the "unreached" through decentralization of planning and management systems. In recent years the country has also been able to shift the focus from expansion to improvement of quality of services.	Targeting with information from local governments on population needs
Democratic People's Republic of Korea	All the health establishments are run as public and state responsibilities.	Examples of collaboration across public agencies not available for this report.
India	The National Rural Health Mission, launched in 2005, aims to provide accessible, affordable and accountable quality health services even to the poorest households in the remotest rural regions.	Negotiation with finance and development for budget and health equity as part of overall development
Indonesia	Indonesia has significantly scaled-up coverage and accessibility of essential health services through establishing a financial medium. The Government launched an initiative to develop "Alert Villages" (Desa Siaga) nationwide.	Coordination and planning with district governments
Maldives	The Government of Maldives has expanded curative services to establish a multi-level referral system, which is more decentralized and has greater NGO and private sector involvement in service delivery. Efforts are also being made to establish a social security system, which includes basic health care and encourages individual organizations to establish mechanisms for covering the health expenses of their employees.	Mediating the involvement of industrial and economic sectors and their stakeholders in designing policy
Myanmar	Myanmar has given high priority to developing an adequate number of workforces of qualified health personnel. To ensure equity in health care and reduce discrepancies between different geographical areas, new universities have been opened in Central and Upper Myanmar.	Negotiating the associated education and workforce policies
Nepal	The government is: (a) working to make essential health care services available to all people through primary health care centres, (b) trying to decentralize health systems management to encourage greater people participation, (c) trying to promote and facilitate public-private/NGO partnerships in the delivery of health services, and (d) making efforts to improve the quality of health care through total quality management of human, financial and physical resources.	Working through local government to ensure appropriate human resources, physical infrastructure and participation mechanisms
Sri Lanka	Sri Lanka has been able to scale-up accessibility and coverage of primary health care. To tackle the increasing problem of non-communicable diseases, the Ministry of Health will lead in planning and sponsoring a major national behaviour change communication programme and set off activities aimed at healthy lifestyle changes in targeted population groups. It will be carried out through intersectoral and multisectoral collaboration with relevant departments and agencies.	Addressing differential exposure and vulnerability through collaborating with other sectors to shape values, social norms and information availability and sharing
Thailand	Recent initiatives in strengthening primary health care include: (a) giving primary care centres a new look through renovation, refurbishment of physical structure of public health facilities with adequate supply of medical and non-medical equipment, establishment of some public primary care centres with full-time physicians and involvement of private clinics by using the financing mechanism of the 30 Baht scheme; (b) increasing competency of health personnel at primary care centres through upgrading the General Practitioner Residency Training Programme to Family Physician Training Programme; (c) establishment of Referral Coordinating Centre (RCC) to manage referral systems effectively and providing financial incentives to hospitals that provide reserve beds for admissions; and (d) integrating community-based preventive and health promotion and Thai traditional medicine in primary care centres.	Working across national government and through local government to ensure training, infrastructure and participation mechanisms for involvement and empowerment
Timor-Leste	The Government has adopted a policy of integrating health systems with other sectors, targeting groups to achieve the greatest health impacts, developing policies on human resources for health, appropriate to the needs of the country, promoting access to basic health care for vulnerable groups, mainstreaming gender health concerns in all programmes, and working with relevant sectors/organizations to advocate an improved status for women by promoting equal rights for men and women in access to care.	Addressing gender norms in government and in society through design of policies and services

Source: Adapted from WHO Regional Conference on Revitalizing Primary Health Care (WHO 2009), as summarized by Pandav (2012), commissioned by WHO-SEARO, September 2012

Ministry of Physical Planning and Works, Ministry of Agriculture and Cooperatives, Ministry of Education, and Ministry of Local Development and Social Protection played roles providing interventions for targeted populations.

3.2 Prevention and control of the global burden of specific diseases

A number of countries in South-East Asia have been addressing the control of both communicable and noncommunicable diseases using an intersectoral or multisectoral approach and in so doing, touched upon action in several areas of determinants of health. Joint departmental committees and intersectoral/multisectoral national committees exist in many disease control programmes, particularly under the major global programmes such as HIV/AIDS, malaria, tuberculosis and noncommunicable diseases.

With regard to infectious diseases, the intersectoral approach has been adopted under national strategies to reduce the stigma of tuberculosis and address social determinants of health related to the disease. Multisectoral taskforces have been formed with representatives across ministries, local governments, and NGOs to control HIV/AIDS in almost all the countries where national HIV/AIDS control programmes were formulated. For example, in Bhutan, the National HIV/AIDS Commission responsible for policy-making and the Multisectoral Task Force responsible for implementation were formulated with intersectoral cooperation from the Ministry of Health, Ministry of Education, police and armed forces, municipalities, and non-governmental organizations. These multisectoral taskforces in HIV/AIDS and tuberculosis have been successful in raising awareness communication, advocacy, social mobilization for public policy and behavioural changes.

Intersectoral teams for water safety and waste management have contributed a great deal to disease control nation-wide, particularly in countries such as Bangladesh, Bhutan, and Nepal. Coordination between water and health authorities brought not only improvement of water quality, but also capacity building for coordination, empowering communities and families, improving infrastructure, reducing burden of diseases and improving maternal and child health.

Recently, with the United Nations Political Declaration of the High Level Meeting of the General Assembly on the Prevention and Control of Non-Communicable Diseases (2011), the Member States and international community were requested to take considerable action to integrate measures to prevent noncommunicable diseases into their national development agendas. Multisectoral actions through Health in All Policies and a whole-of-government approach were called for. Thus, the HiAP approach and multisectoral actions have been adopted throughout the process of development of national plans of actions for NCD control and prevention in countries of the South-East Asia Region. A number of countries now have national steering committees or commissions for prevention and control of noncommunicable diseases. In Indonesia, the National NCD Network and National Strategic Plan provides an overarching umbrella for intersectoral/multisectoral actions with clear roles and responsibilities of all partners. In Sri Lanka and Bhutan, the national policy and strategic framework became the guiding principle for intersectoral/multisectoral actions. Thailand's integrative Healthy Lifestyle Strategic Plan (2011–2020) provides the framework for intersectoral/multisectoral actions at national and subnational levels.

Mainstreaming of healthy lifestyles in health promoting schools and healthy settings has been adopted in almost all countries in the South-East Asia Region. Healthy settings were already intersectoral/multisectoral in nature and thus could easily be tapped into for further development of a Health in All Policies approach to prevention and control of diseases and their determinants, both communicable and noncommunicable.

3.3 Risk factors (tobacco and alcohol consumption, food safety, injuries and road safety)

The **Tobacco Free Initiative** is a prominent programme in the region and drives the development of several multisectoral actions, including legislative frameworks to ensure that all relevant partners are making concerted efforts to control the use of tobacco, ban advertisement and counter tobacco industries. Almost all of the countries in the South-East Asia Region have legislation banning the sale of tobacco to minors, while some countries have banned tobacco use in public places and in government institutions.

The WHO Framework Convention on Tobacco Control (FCTC) is an important international instrument that lays out the legal commitments of Member States, triggering national and subnational tobacco control committees, task forces and initiatives in countries. Schools, youth, NGOs and networks of advocates play important roles in the process. Among countries in South-East Asia, Bhutan, India and Thailand have shown strong government support of implementation of the WHO FCTC using a whole-of-government approach.

Generally WHO FCTC legislation and policies prescribe the use of pictorial warning messages on tobacco packages, ban sale of tobacco to minors, ban tobacco advertisement, and ban smoking in public places, educational institutions, and office spaces. Smoke-free public places, schools, cities and workplaces have been implemented through multisectoral collaboration, particularly with ministries of health, justice, information, education, transportation, tourism, city authorities and local administrations, along with the media for campaigns and public support.

In Bhutan, despite the long history of anti-tobacco practices as part of the Buddhist culture, tobacco products were readily available during the 1980s and 1990s. Coupled with no legal restrictions, this contributed to a rise in the sale and consumption of tobacco in the country. The launch of the WHO FCTC at the World Health Assembly in May 2003 was a turning point at which the Royal Government of Bhutan made a firm commitment to be the first country to be tobacco free. At the Eighty-second Session of National Assembly, the government reached a consensus to impose a nationwide ban on tobacco sales and prohibit smoking in all public places, endorsing the ratification of the WHO FCTC. The whole country took effective action from 17 December 2004 with a series of multisectoral stakeholder meetings. The Royal Government of Bhutan was able to identify sectors responsible for control of tobacco use, create an enforcement team, monitor tobacco flow at all ports of entry, enforce penalties for failing to comply with regulations, increase tax, and control tobacco smuggling, as well as draft the First Tobacco Control Bill in 2007. In June 2010, the Tobacco Control Act was enacted, and provides a comprehensive ban on the advertisement, promotion, and sponsorship of tobacco and tobacco products, restricting appearance of tobacco products in all domestic media. The Act mandates the state to carry out comprehensive activities to advocate and educate the public, as well as enforce the rules and regulations and adhere to the Act through multisectoral cooperation at all levels (Rinchen, 2013).

The Government of India was one of the first eight countries to ratify the WHO FCTC in 2004. The National Tobacco Control Programme roll out of the WHO FCTC from the beginning of the 11th Five Year Plan in 2007–2008 was implemented in 21 out of 35 States/Union Territories in the country. The National Tobacco Control Cell was established in the Ministry of Health and Family Welfare responsible for overall policy formulation, planning, monitoring, and evaluation of the activities envisaged under the National Tobacco Control Programme. The National Tobacco Control Cell is a high-level intersectoral committee consisting of an inter-ministerial task force from 11 ministries at national level. Additional authorities, civil society, and representatives from state-level government are special invitees to the task force. Coordination between sectors is reinforced by ongoing sensitization activities (trainings and workshops at national, regional, and state levels) led by the health sector. Stakeholders across all sectors play important roles in raising awareness, controlling and banning public smoking, providing anti-tobacco education in schools, ensuring health warnings on all tobacco products, mobilizing communities and representing the voice of tobacco victims.

In Thailand, the National Committee for the Control of Tobacco Use, established in 1989, plays an important role as a policy-coordinating mechanism. It consists of the

Permanent Secretaries of related ministries, representatives of civil society, and prominent experts on tobacco control. The committee is responsible for drafting policy and guidelines on tobacco control, cooperating with different organizations on tobacco control activities, and accelerating, controlling, monitoring, and evaluating the legal enforcement of notifications issued by the Ministry of Public Health. Within the Ministry of Public Health, there is the Tobacco Control Cluster under the Department of Diseases Control, working together with all the relevant departments and units, controlling risk factors for alcohol consumption, as well as mental health. The Tobacco Control Cluster is coordinated by the Ministry of Public Health with other departments and ministries outside health, such as the Excise Department and the Customs Department, Ministry of Finance, Office of Royal Thai Police, Office of the Prime Minister, Department of Special Investigation, Ministry of Justice, Public Relations Department, Ministry of Education, provincial and local administration, and NGOs. The Thai Health Promotion Foundation is another strong mechanism for social mobilization, social marketing, and financial support to tobacco control activities in Thailand. Major successes have been attributed to having intersectoral coordinating mechanisms at the highest level with national bodies and support for the social mobilization implementation and monitoring process.

Multisectoral/intersectoral strategies have been used in **interventions to reduce the harmful use of alcohol** in the Region. From the literature review in 2012 (Pandav, 2012), this was found to be the case in Bhutan, India, Sri Lanka, and Thailand. Most of the existing evidence showed that the countries' interventions were mainly focused on protecting health, by reducing exposure to risk factors and environments, without clear strategies designed to promote health through intersectoral partnerships. In Bhutan, interventions to reduce the harmful use of alcohol were implemented through regulations, licensing and enforcement, education, and treatment focusing on community actions, for example, alcohol is strictly prohibited in social gatherings, and fines are enforced for drinking in public. With intersectoral cooperation, it is expected that Bhutan will be able to reduce the harmful use of alcohol. In India, the intersectoral/multisectoral actions to reduce harmful use of alcohol have been implemented through cooperation of the Global Road Safety Programme, the National Institute of Mental Health and Neurosciences and the Bangalore City Police, formulated as the Bangalore Agenda Task Force.

The Government of Sri Lanka has implemented a comprehensive package of legislation and administrative measures for reducing consumption of alcohol per capita.

The National Authority on Tobacco and Alcohol, Department of Excise, the police, and the Ministry of Health are key intersectoral bodies involved in implementing the Tobacco and Alcohol Act 2006. The legislation bans direct and indirect advertisement and promotion of alcohol products, including sponsorships by the alcohol industry. A series of alcohol prohibition measures consists of the prohibition of the sale of alcohol for persons under the age of 21, sale through vending machines, free distribution, public consumption, sale on religious holidays, and a requirement that all the distributors/sale points need licences. The implementations were carried out through coordination between multiple government agencies, namely education, police, justice, media, trade and commerce, and sports.

Thailand has a long history of controlling the use of alcohol, beginning in 1950. The Liquor Act B.E. 2493 (1950) regulates taxation of alcohol and licenses sale outlets. Many legislation and policy interventions have been put in place, but there was an inconsistency of implementation and enforcement. However, recent social movements to reduce the harmful use of alcohol in Thailand were contributed to by the Thai Health Promotion Foundation, which saw the support of multisectoral actions to reduce alcohol use and other risk factors. The Alcohol and Beverage Control Act B.E. 2551 (2008) provided more structural interventions and prevention and control at national and provincial levels. The Act contains regulations on marketing, physical availability of alcohol, and drinking venues, where multisectoral agencies are responsible for ensuring effective measures.

Nutrition and food safety initiatives in the South-East Asia Region showed strong commitment and

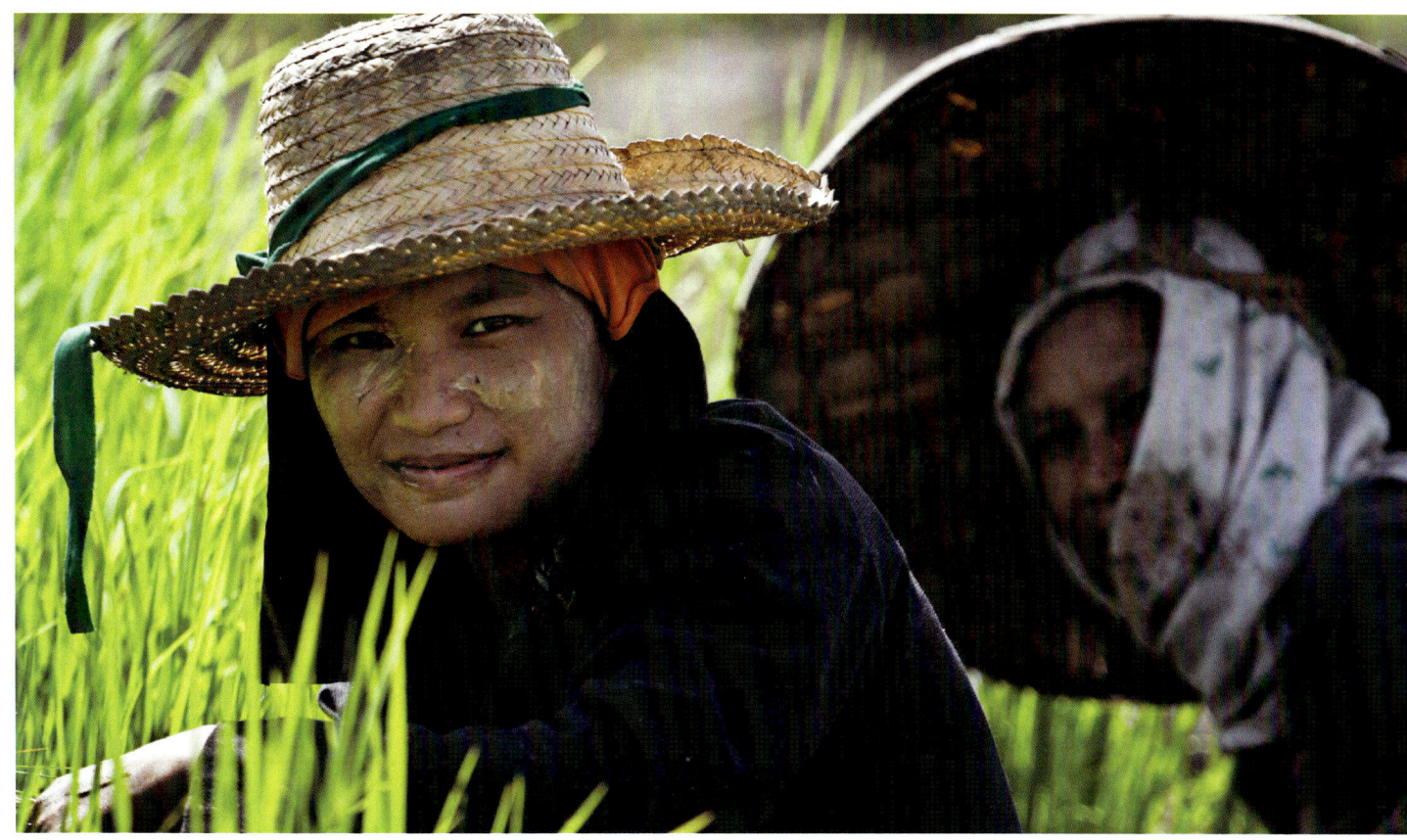

Rice famers look on as they prepare plants in a field. ©David Longstreath/IRIN

needs for intersectoral mechanisms and actions addressing malnutrition, food safety, and social factors. A call for action in the Bi-regional Meeting on Scaling Up Nutrition, held in Colombo, Sri Lanka, in August 2011, included strengthening the multisectoral approach with a focus on inequity, vulnerable groups, and inclusiveness in social protection schemes. Nutrition-related challenges in the Region continue to be issues of child malnutrition, micronutrient deficiencies,coupled with overweight and obesity due to lifestyle changes, availability of imported and processed food, and aggressive marketing for unhealthy products. Food security measures to ensure availability and affordability for the poor, children and neglected populations, particularly women and the elderly are being implemented through multisectoral collaboration with a wide range of ministries in some countries. In India and Nepal, for example, the national nutrition programmes emphasise maternal protection and an income safety net programme. However, the multisectoral programmes for nutrition and food security in the Region still need to be strengthened for effective coordination at all levels.

The Multisectoral Nutrition Programme that was established in Nepal in 2012, following a recognized string of multisectoral nutrition initiatives since the 1970s. Integrated Rural Development projects such as Rasuwa Nuwakot Integrated Rural Development and Mahakali Integrated Rural Development in the 1970s built on a holistic approach to development, which attempted to address multiple constraints simultaneously through appropriate planning for development priorities. Development areas of focus included health and nutrition, agriculture, education, and rural roads. A nutrition coordination committee was established as a result of these processes in the National Planning Commission in 1977. The Multisectoral Nutrition Programme was initiated, which focused on specific interventions, such as improving feeding, care practices in the health sector, and nutrition-sensitive interventions for families and communities. Nutrition-sensitive interventions included actions that are led by other sectors, comprising those aimed at addressing food availability, affordability, access, and quality of food. A multisectoral planning framework was used to define strategic objectives, interventions, expected outputs, estimated budget, and monitoring indicators for each sector. The planning framework, coupled with existing decentralized governance structure under the mandate of the Local Self Governance Act (1999), included expansion of infrastructure for public health, education, and agriculture. With multiple sectors involved, and a wide concept of health interventions comprising nutrition-sensitive interventions, the Multisectoral Nutrition Programme provides a current window of opportunity for the institutionalization of Health in All Policies in Nepal.

The 2012 Food and Nutritional Security Policy in Bhutan recognized the multisectoral actions needed for food and nutrition security. The High-level Food and Nutrition Security Committee was thus initiated to coordinate effective policy planning and implementation, to provide strategic direction for effective intersectoral communication and policy coordination, to promote and synergize different departments and ministries. The Gross National Happiness Commission (GNHC) acts as a secretariat for high-level food and nutrition security.

Ten out of 11 Member States in the South-East Asia Region established national-level multisectoral bodies with dedicated focal agencies to review the national food safety policies. Legislation related to food safety, particularly on street food, has been issued in countries such as Bangladesh, the Democratic People's Republic of Korea, India, Indonesia, Myanmar, Sri Lanka and Thailand. Ministries of health play important roles in providing technical supervision to non-health sectors to promote food safety and the implementation of national policies and laws, particularly the ministries of agriculture, home affairs, education, employment, social welfare, transportation, city management, department of development, national and sub-national local authorities, and non-governmental organizations. Street food networks are an example of successful food safety interventions, which promote health in non-health sector policies.

Prevention of injuries and road safety is a good example of the need for intersectoral actions in most countries of the South-East Asia Region that impact policies and plans in other sectors. Leading road safety agencies lie outside the ministry of health. While coordination agencies for national road safety exist in Bangladesh, Sri Lanka and Thailand, not all have clear connections and links to health. Ministries of transportation and communication in these countries have autonomous functions in enforcing existing legislation and operations. In some countries, there are joint responsibilities between the ministry of transport and communication, and the police department. In Bhutan, road safety has been adopted in the Bhutan Decade Plan for Road Safety Action 2012–2022, which requires collaboration from several partners, including ministries of health, works and human settlement, road and transportation, information and communications, education, and the Royal Bhutan Police.

Few countries have established intersectoral mechanisms between health and transport and where they do exist, they are at the operational level. In India, intersectoral actions take place between the Ministry of Health and Family Welfare and the Ministry of Road, Transport and Highways. In Delhi, emergency medical service systems are linked to the centralized accident and trauma services society, which was formed by the Delhi City Administration. Under the 11th Five Year Plan, the Government of India launched the National Highways Accident Relief Services Scheme. The States/Union Territories and NGOs provided first aid and transferal of road accident victims to the nearest facility.

In Thailand, the Road Safety Operating Centre plays a leading role in road safety, operated under the Department of Disaster Prevention and Mitigation by the Ministry of Interior. However, in Thailand, road safety initiatives were started by the Ministry of Health, which later was linked to prevention of drunk driving, and warnings on the adverse effects of alcohol on health.

3.4 Health promotion and healthy public policies

National health promotion policies and master plans in several countries have used the development of a "healthy vision" as a guiding principle to promote healthy behaviour and call for intersectoral and multisectoral actions. Some countries have made progress toward establishing mechanisms that enable public policies to take health considerations into account, ensuring that the impact of the policies improves the population's health.

Multisectoral partners promoting healthy behaviour vary depending on the settings within the national and subnational contexts. Health promotion has advocated multisectoral actions for more than two decades. The Bangkok Declaration for Health Promotion in 2005 addressed global determinants of health with "All for Health". All for Health is an aspiration by the health sector for other sectors of government and society to contribute further to population health. Active health promotion in schools, hospitals, communities, workplaces and cities plays an important role in raising health concerns among the public as mentioned previously. Some collaborative efforts are made across sectors. Schools and hospitals promoting health and healthy cities are the key settings for successful implementation, which has depended on a wide range of partners from other sectors.

In the Maldives, health promotion is integrated in the country's 7th National Development Plan, the Health Master Plan 2006–2015, and Vision 2020. Healthy setting projects encompass health promoting schools, health promoting hospitals, and healthy islands where multisectoral partnerships and collaboration are practiced.

As practiced in many countries in the Region, a number of school health programmes are implemented by national committees or through national policies which coordinate and implement school health activities with intersectoral partners, especially between the ministries of education and health. However, in some countries these programmes are implemented and coordinated by more than two or three ministries, making them multisectoral in nature. For example, in Myanmar the National School Health Committee was established at central government level along with school health committees at the state, division, district, township, and school levels. These committees are composed of representatives from the ministries of health, education, social welfare, indigenous medicine, sports and physical education, city development, and local NGOs. In India, the Ministry of Health and Family Welfare takes the lead on school health policy and programmes however implementation is carried out by multistakeholders from sectors other than health.

In Sri Lanka, the Ministries of Health and of Education have joint responsibility for the School Health Promotion Programme. Each ministry also has a coordination unit to ensure its collaboration goes as planned. The National School Health Promotion Committee is constituted of the Steering Committee with line ministries from different sectors. The Committee is responsible for formulating national policies on school health promotion, evaluating and monitoring the activities relevant to school health promotion and providing necessary feedback for successful programme implementation. Multisectoral coordinating bodies for school health promotion in Sri Lanka also exist at all levels from national and provincial, to a district and zonal school health promotion committees and a School Health Promotion Advisory Committee.

In Indonesia, the National Coordinating Board for the School Health Programme was established with representatives from the ministries of health, education, religious affairs, and internal affairs, while provincial board members are varied within a local context. The city or district may have the District Mayor of the City chair the District/City Coordination Board, which gives guidance to operational boards for activities at every school level. However, these coordinating boards may not receive the level of support required from their centralized bodies at ministerial level because of the decentralized structure of these authorities.

In Thailand, the school health programme is primarily the responsibility of the Ministry of Public Health. However, health activities are included in school curriculums and policies. Intersectoral activities for the school health programme are mostly at operational level. There is no designated health promotion unit or school health programme focal point in the Ministry of Education.

Beyond the establishment of intersectoral mechanisms and ad hoc campaigns for social mobilization, further understanding of how the past multisectoral/intersectoral actions for health and on their determinants raises health concerns to policy-makers in other sectors was needed for healthy public policies.

In Thailand, **health impact assessment (HIA)** has been an important tool and an entry point for healthy public policies. The National Health Act clearly states the rights of an individual or a group of people to request impact evaluations and to participate in the evaluation of public policy (National Health Act 2007, Section 11). People should have access to information, explanations, and underlying reasons prior to approval being granted for a policy or activity which may affect their health or the health of a community, and shall have the right to formally express their opinions on such matters. Health impact assessment in Thailand has been implemented under the healthy public policies concept which was started in 2000. It has become a mechanism for the whole health system reform, in which public policies of all sectors are accountable and contribute to health of the whole population.

During the development of Thailand's Health Constitution, debates emphasized the role of public participation. The Thai Constitution 2007 Section 67 also states that *"... any project or activity which may cause serious impacts on the environment, natural resources, and health, cannot proceed without an impact assessment addressing environmental quality, and the health of populations in affected communities, and such an assessment must include a public hearing process for affected people and stakeholders. ... The public is entitled to sue any governmental agency failing to comply with these principles."*

However, despite having legislation and constitutional support for the application of HIA in Thailand, the institutional structure of HIA itself does not require a specific institute or administrative body. It has become a "social mechanism" that stakeholders in all sectors can use to protect and support the rights and the health of Thai people, applying a participatory approach to healthy public policy. After a decade of experience in Thailand, the HIA process has been sustained through people empowerment, along with technical support from academic, and political, as well as legislative support from the National Health Act, whereby the National Health Commission played an important role. Today, in Thailand, the HIA network is strong and has expanded to include stakeholders from a range of other sectors, growing beyond Thailand's borders and out and across the Region.

3.5 Intersectoral actions addressing determinants of health

In 2005, the WHO Commission on Social Determinants of Health visited countries in South-East Asia and the WHO Regional Office for South-East Asia organized a regional consultation on social determinants of health in Delhi, India, which clearly led the beginning of the discussion on health equity in all policies in the South-East Asia Region. Subsequently, the Region developed the "Colombo Call for Action" (2009) and funding was provided to the "Light House Project" in Sri Lanka, aimed at addressing social determinants of health through a broad range of actions. Under this Project, a number of case studies and projects were commissioned to understand the social determinants of health in rural, urban and estate settings. Research studies were also commissioned to look at the access to care issues during an Acute Coronary Syndrome and the cost burden of Diabetes Mellitus at household level, and on the health system. The economic burden to patients undergoing treatment for diabetes mellitus in relation to travel, food and other indirect costs, as well as lost income was estimated to assess barriers to care. Pilot projects included tackling mental illness in the former post-conflict zone in the Northern provinces, gender-based violence, and interventions for dengue fever in Colombo Municipal Areas. (WHO 2012). A key outcome of the project was a comprehensive checklist to guide dengue investigations was developed including social determinants. Finally, a PHC-based model for NCD prevention, involving training of pre-school teachers and parents on noncommunicable disease prevention and other discrete activities for health with district government and

NGOs, was developed in one area with a view to replication in other areas.

Similarly, in the Maldives, a study on *"Social Disparities in Health in the Maldives: an Assessment and Implications"* was commissioned by WHO-SEARO to examine intersectoral actions required to tackle disparities in health. The study also recommended strengthening research and health information systems to collect reliable data for informed policy-making and emphasized the importance of the role of the state in financing and delivery of health care, especially for the prevention and control of NCDs.

Among Member States of the South-East Asia Region, the health system reform in Thailand is cited as an example for providing a platform for intersectoral actions to address social determinants of health in various health activities. According to the National Health Act 2007, "health assembly" is defined as a process in which the public and related government agencies exchange their knowledge and learn from each other through a systematic forum of public participations that lead to suggestions or resolutions for healthy public policies to improve health of the population. Health assembly can be organized at different levels national, area-based, local-based, etc. The National Health Assembly (NHA) was established to serve as a public space for active engagement by all sectors and stakeholders, including civil society. The process of NHA generates a "soft power" and provides a "social space" for stakeholders in policy engagement.[1] Almost 70–80% of agendas of all the National Health Assemblies in Thailand address issues related to determinants of health and call for policy accountability and actions beyond health sectors. For example, the needs of disabled people have been addressed through the provision of legal rights and social mobilization, as have issues of environmental protection, community livelihood and control of pesticides.

The National Rural Health Mission, India's flagship health programme recognizes the role of social determinants of health such as drinking water, female literacy, nutrition, early childhood development, sanitation, and women's empowerment, and seeks to adopt a convergent approach under the umbrella of the district plan. The thrust of the Mission is on establishing a fully functional, community owned, decentralized health delivery system with intersectoral convergence at all levels, to ensure simultaneous action on a wide range of determinants of health, such as access to water, sanitation, education, nutrition, and social and gender equality (Pandav, 2012).

Timor-Leste is classified as a fragile state, which is transitioning from a phase of internal security to the next development phase of state building to newly established systems of national governance. The United Nations Mission in Timor-Leste has been the core support for country development from 2002–2012. The country is still in the process of formulating policies and legislation. The intent for intersectoral actions has been expressed in national and health policy documents. A recent study (Pandav, 2013) commissioned by WHO Regional Office for South-East Asia found that the first National Development Plan of Timor-Leste indicated the Vision for 2020 focusing on agriculture, education, health, and infrastructure development. The Timor-Leste Strategic Development Plan 2011–2030 envisions three key priorities for development, namely social capital, infrastructure, and economic development. The Strategic Development Plan is an integrated package of strategic policies which clearly identifies the roles of other sectors in improving health. Health is an important component of social capital for a start. The agricultural sector plays a role in tackling issues of food efficiency, increasing livestock production and fisheries, as well as activities that will enable more diversified and nutritionally balanced diets for the population. Infrastructure initiatives are involved in the provision of electric systems and sustainable energies that also contribute to reduction of indoor pollution from traditional cooking. The housing and development sector would seek to provide better housing facilities, and decrease overcrowding in households, in order to reduce airborne and transmissible diseases. Improving education and literacy is key to tackling socioeconomic determinants of health with access to appropriate information (Pandav, 2013).

---

[1] Tipicha Posayanonda, Nattaya Thaennin, Orapan Srisookwatana (2012) *Thailand's National Health Assembly: Intersectoral Action for Health.* Commissioned by WHO-SEARO, Funded by WHO-Kobe Center, December 2012.

4. FOSTERING FACTORS, BUILDING BLOCKS, AND DRIVERS FOR IMPLEMENTATION OF HIAP

The approach to Health in All Policies remains an inspiration and ideology without, as yet, clear indicators, criteria, or benchmarks to measure progress on implementation. Formulating a clearer understanding of the building blocks for applying the Health in All Policies approach will be crucial in the coming years.

Over the decades, Member States of the South-East Asian Region have gone through a series of national health reforms and decentralization, which shifted the power structure within the countries. The role of the health sector in each country varies according to their different sociopolitical contexts. High-level political engagement in health and public policies is not always explicit in most countries. An existing national mechanism for high-level development plans, such as the Gross National Happiness Commission, National Planning Commissions, National Social and Economic Development Board, United Nations Country Team and the United Nations Development/Partnership Frameworks (UNDAF/UNPAF) can play significant roles and may effectively address health/quality of life of the population beyond the health sector and ensure multisectoral responses, coordination, and support.

Leadership and governance structures need to be in place to ensure commitment from the highest level decision-makers, who can direct solutions to tackle structural determinants of health associated with government sectors overall. Countries in the South-East Asia Region have different levels of intersectoral actions. Some are at the highest level of a national government policy-setting body, some are middle-range of ministerial and standing committees, and some are at the implementation level. Windows of opportunity to address health concerns using the HiAP approach were found throughout all levels, including as part of the national development plan, building cooperation with international communities, and developing partnership frameworks, such as a partnership for the Millennium Development Goals (MDGs), the post-2015 development agenda, or for specific programmes, like the Global Fund for Malaria, Tuberculosis and HIV/AIDS. It was important that these efforts be built upon existing mechanisms and governance structures, which fostered support to help achieve goals.

4.1 Creating opportunities and driving forces

The MDGs were one of the first development agendas in which Member States made significant efforts to take intersectoral actions to address not only health concerns, but also other development factors. From regional and country consultations in South-East Asia, it was found that the MDGs were an important driving force for the national development plan and policies, in which many sectors could work together for the same goals with a shared amount of responsibility and resources. With existing UN country teams who work and coordinate activities within the **UN Development Framework (UNDAF)** or UN Partnership Framework (UNPAF), countries consider the mechanism to be most useful, particularly where there have been resource constraints. The next opportunity for countries to strategically put health concerns in all policies will be in the post-2015 development agenda and the new cycle of the national development plan.

Some countries in South-East Asia created their own opportunity to promote health beyond health care and medicine through **national health reform**, such as in Thailand through a participatory process of drafting the National Health Act. Social mobilization for health system reform in Thailand caused a paradigm shift in the health sector and beyond with broad definitions going beyond physical and psychological health to include social and spiritual health. It called upon stakeholders across sectors to manage health and tackle determinants of health in a coordinated fashion. The National Health Act was a tool for social empowerment and changing the mindset of the health profession and other sectors. The whole society needed to act and become accountable for and contribute to the health of the entire country.

Other countries such as Indonesia, Nepal and Sri Lanka and some parts of States in India utilized opportunities through **decentralization of government structure** to make an effort with intersectoral actions. The role of communities, grass-root organizations and local government has significantly contributed to coordination and collaboration between state government and all sectors. Local authorities have different models of decentralization to use their power and resources to enable people in communities and facilitate government officials and experts to support intersectoral actions taking place in a local context. Healthy communities, healthy municipalities and healthy districts are examples of a subnational achievement to make health the centre of development and create common goals so all sectors can take action for a better health outcome. A Health in All Policies approach could be implemented in subnational policies, such as those of urban and all local administration, etc. Although at the beginning the decentralization was for political more than managerial reasons, in the long term, it assumed local responsibility, accountability, and self-sufficiency elements. Human resources and capacities have been problematic, and continue to be a concern in many countries in the Region.

In India, **the social protection platform and flagship programme for vulnerable populations,** such as the National Rural Health Mission, is one of the driving forces bringing intersectoral action to address the health of the poor, vulnerable population and determinants of health.

4.2 Legislative framework

Legislative frameworks such as constitutions, national health acts, tobacco control law or road safety acts, can influence public policies at all levels to take health and its determinants into consideration. For example, the Constitution of the Kingdom of Thailand (2007) and National Health Act (2007) indicate that health impact assessment can be requested by the people and must be practiced in all policy development processes, particularly when the development programmes have a high potential impact on the health of population.

After several legislative frameworks created for the specific control of health risk factors, such as anti-tobacco laws, following the WHO FCTC, it was found that there was cooperation and collaboration on intersectoral policies. Specific legislative responses to controlling health risks offered an important opportunity for countries to pull together and tackle specific health issues using the whole-of-government approach.

However, the health sector is not yet sensitized to recognize many areas of opportunities, such as poverty reduction, social protection, and sustainable development where the health sector could actively participate in the policy development process, even though it does not always have full capacity to approach the notion of working with other agencies, particularly in social and economic sectors. An understanding of the politics of policy-making and the policy development process is required, in order to be able to recognize the appropriate entry points and how best to make useful and strategic contributions to other sectors and vice versa. The issue of transparency and accountability in South-East Asian countries needs to be further strengthened through various procedures and measures. If ways to monitor and evaluate were built into public policies and plans, this could enhance the accountability of intersectoral/

multisectoral actions. A reporting system and public hearings, as part of transparency and accountability, have not been institutionalized in most countries.

4.3 Institutional intersectoral mechanism

Several institutional intersectoral mechanisms exist in countries in the South East Asia Region; however, most of the mechanisms are aimed at operational coordination. The highest level of intersectoral mechanisms for policy development is with the parliamentary/cabinet or the national committees, in which the prime minister or president is the chairman. The body of an intersectoral mechanism may consist of all line ministries or concerned ministries, but lead agencies assigned to their core functions are responsible for the different agendas. Without vision or political will to use a systematic and whole-of-government approach, the committee may not actively engage other sectors to think about issues of the concerned sectors. In almost all countries, the ministry of health, in general, is not the most politically and economically powerful. There is a need for strong leadership and technical support to show the political, social and economic impact of policies and actions across sectors on health issues.

Some high-level mechanisms in countries in the Region are ad hoc in nature, thus sustainability could hinder efforts made from one government to the other when a political party and structure changes. Government policies and mandates are often operated without accountability, or policy auditing. Public participation and the ability for the media to question political accountability are limited.

4.4 Joint/innovative financial mechanism

Collaboration and coordination mechanisms are necessary for intersectoral governance initiatives, and joint-government development programmes and targets. Past experiences in countries in South-East Asia show that joint financial mechanisms are limited and rarely visible. The parliament or cabinet in most cases instructs responsible agencies to provide resources to take action on the priorities. In few circumstances, a special budget could be allocated to the ministry of health to take the lead in collaboration with other sectors and share the resources when health concerns such as HIV/AIDS and polio eradication become a national agenda. Some issues on social determinants of health were allocated to other sector ministries. For example, the Ministry of Labour implemented and funded a pilot project to train traditional tobacco rollers for alternative vocations as part of intersectoral actions under the National Development Council for National Tobacco and Cigarette Control in India.

Innovative financial mechanisms evidenced in the Region are the conditional cash transfer programmes in India and Bangladesh, and tobacco taxation in Thailand. The report on the Ten-Year Review of the Thai Health Promotion Foundation (2001–2011) showed the success of awareness-raising by generating interest in health issues, not only in individuals, but also in communities, and private organizations, as well as ministries and parliament. The funds from the Thai Health Promotion Foundation had been allocated to health promotion across sectors and multistakeholders who contributed to achieving healthy public policies and, potentially moving towards achieving "health" in all policies. Concerted efforts in sharing responsibilities and joint-funding coordination are key factors for sustaining effective management of a Health in All Policies approach.

4.5 Capacity and human resources

In the South-East Asia Region, the quality and capacity of human resources for intersectoral work varies. Although the countries have been practising intersectoral action, cooperation and coordination for some time, bringing together the elements contained in the Health in All Policies approach (HiAP), which includes more systematic accountability for health impacts in policy-making across diverse sectors, with a determinants focus, is a rather unfamiliar concept. Thus, the capacity of individuals and institutions to implement the approach in South-East Asia is limited. A few examples of intersectoral experiences that led to healthy public policies were seen in the health impact

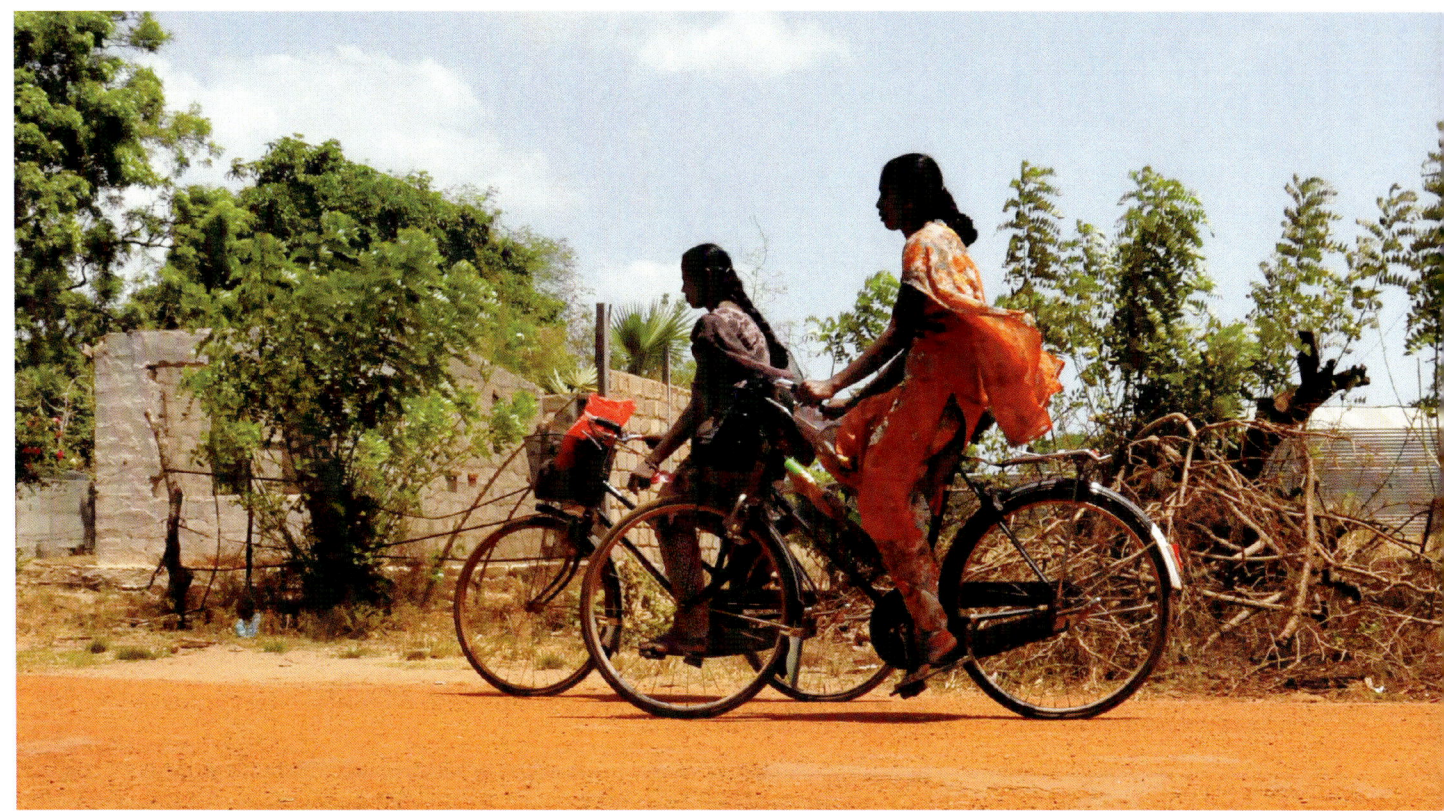

Women riding bicycles along a main road in Sri Lanka. ©Amantha Perera/IRIN

assessment practices in Thailand. It took Thailand more than a decade to create a critical mass and empower people, communities, and societies to be aware of how policies, projects, and incidents (such as flood, disaster, gas pipe leaks, etc.) may impact negatively on health. Health impact assessment in Thailand thereby became an important participatory tool to empower people and build the capacity of organizations to work across sectors.

More can be learnt from Thailand. Leadership and collaboration skills of health personnel for engaging with other sectors have been important to the success of Thailand's health system reform process. Prior to the launch of the National Health Act 2007, the Health System Research Institute expanded technical knowledge beyond the health sector using the new paradigm and social innovation for health to capture linkages between health and other disciplines, particularly economic, social, political, and legislation with holistic and systematic perspectives. Evidence generated by the health sector was presented at a national symposium and simplified for deliberation at health assemblies at different levels. Action research was used for some of the research and the impact research methodology was then translated into practical solutions and used to guide policy change through a participatory process. The process was initiated as knowledge management which was brought to the attention of policy-makers. Through social mobilization, the health issues became national and local agendas and there was a call for all sectors to take action. The example of Thailand may be unique, however, it showed leadership by bringing together three factors to bring about change, the so-called "triangle of power": knowledge (technical), social movement (health assemblies) and advocacy (media), and political power (policy-makers).

In many countries, the capacity to mobilize resources and intersectoral actions lies in an individual engaging in the programme/projects at different levels of administrations or bureaucracies, and their gaining political will. There is currently no clear institutional capacity in the region. Sustainability of intersectoral actions suffers when the staff turnover rate is high or rotates to different offices. The type of capacity and human resources necessary for sustained processes of intersectoral actions across diverse issues and sectors was not seen in most countries in the South-East Asia Region.

5. IMPACTS AND LESSONS LEARNED

5.1 Political will and process

From regional case studies, it can be seen that the political will to take intersectoral actions at policy level and consideration for using Health in All Policies depends on the central governments' interest and the cost or economic implication of the health issue for government finance. Tobacco control and NCDs are major public concerns that gave rise to economic debates for several governments in South-East Asia. Case studies on tobacco control in India and Bhutan showed that the intersectoral actions went beyond the health sector because of the political will from the central government. The effects of tobacco on people's health and livelihood (tobacco growers) are examples that mostly effect the poor and vulnerable populations. The economic gains from tobacco production and costs of providing health care were some of the arguments that central government had to consider, particularly when the government's expenditure on health care was caused by chronic illness due to tobacco use, and other NCDs. The identified ministries, such as agriculture, education, transportation, local government and finance came together to make a concerted effort to ensure the success of tobacco control measures. However, a conflict of interest and the struggles of power and economics were major obstacles. Making the economic case will increasingly be an important area for health to tackle in dealing across government, alongside social mobilization for justice.

Political will for intersectoral actions and implementation of a Health in All Policies approach, including through the whole-of-government approach, has been seen in win-win situations like those created between policy and social sectors in the case of Thailand. National Health Assemblies have demystified health, so that it is not seen as medicine, rather as part of day-to-day activities and the duty of all sectors in the country to take control of, support and ensure that all the population benefits from doing what it can to best promote health. Positive advocacy and the "soft power" process for health in Thailand brought willingness from other sectors to take part, particularly in dealing with social determinants of health. However, rather than from the other sectors, the Thai process experienced (s) some scepticism from the medical profession regarding the power of people and whether the resolutions emerging from national and sub-national health assemblies would have an impact on health.

Intersectoral/multisectoral actions were recognized as an effective approach to provide health interventions for maternal and child health, to control major communicable and noncommunicable diseases, and to promote health at a community level in South-East Asia. Addressing social determinants of health through sectors beyond health was crucial, but less understood by the health sector. As systems progress towards universal health coverage with a commitment to reducing the burden of NCDs, addressing social determinants becomes even more important. Overall, higher potential impacts on health are being observed in policy arenas where health issues are linked with development through health's perspectives and evidence on the social determinants of health and the links with social and health equity.

5.2 Health promotion, health equity and primary health care

In the South-East Asia Region, primary health care and health promotion have a long tradition of working with multisectoral partners to reach the unreached and most vulnerable groups. Revitalization of primary health care in 2008 showed the importance of past successes and addressed the current challenges, especially primary health care in urban setting where pockets of people live without accessibility to quality services. However, the primary prevention and primary care approach that has been practised in South-East Asia somehow lost its broader approach to address public health and determinants of health through health promotion and empowerment at the grass-roots level. Most of the practices focus on health care services at primary health care centres/units and in some cases outreach activities. A study on Health Inequity in the South East Asia Region[1] and a study on urbanization and health (WHO, 2011)[2] revealed a significant need to tackle health challenges through social determinants of health. Health promoting schools, communities, workplaces, hospitals, and healthy cities all contribute with intersectoral/multisectoral actions to this broader, more holistic approach. Healthy city projects such as the Metro-Colombo Urban Development Project,[3] Sri Lanka, is an example of an innovative pilot project addressing social determinants of health through primary health care and citizen participation. Local authorities were able to strengthen the planning process at metropolitan level, support local communities and successfully renew urban infrastructure, by improving sanitation and waste management. The project used both environmental and social impact assessment to address local issues.

In spite of the loss of primary health care focus on social participation and addressing determinants, which is arguably necessary to address health inequities, several examples of country experiences in South-East Asia of using intersectoral actions at the implementation level and to coordinate specific outcomes were found.

Scarcer though were experiences at the policy level. What is clear from the examples cited however was that at the policy level, national intersectoral coordinating bodies report more success more often when the coordinating body is given strategic direction supported by the prime minister, secretary general, or president, as the chairperson so they could guide or direct different departments and ministries to support the policies and programmes. In one way or another, a broad vision of health needs to be an orienting vision for measuring a country's success and sustainable development, as is planned for The post-2015 development Aguda.

5.3 Pragmatic organizational support and social change

Many experiences of countries in the South-East Asia Region have shown that intersectoral actions foster collaboration among different sectors and sometimes between public and private providers. Success of this collaboration lies in sharing a vision and goals but also in sharing information, human and financial resources. Common goals and shared results are important and need to be a joint commitment. Sharing of information, human and financial resources, is one way to support intersectoral actions and to develop effective cooperation across sectors. However, such cooperation is not always sustainable. Often the resources come from the public sector, or centralized bodies that have power to distribute financial and human resources where the issues are politicized. The example of Thailand showed that there were different ways to identify common goals and shared results across a diverse range of sectors, through increasing understanding and changing perspectives on how health is created and who is responsible for the health of the people, through health system reform. The significant paradigm shift on health in Thailand resulted in all the sectors recognizing their roles and contributions to the health of individuals, families, communities, and society, thus the process of health reform between 1998 and 2007. This recognition then led to a series of social change strategies or a mobilization for health and brought about a high level of commitment and sustainability for multisectoral actions through the increased availability of human and financial resources. The National Health Commission, Thai Health Promotion Foundation and

---

1 WHO Regional Office for South-East Asia (2009) *Health Inequities in the South-East Asia Region: Selected Country Case Studies.*
2 WHO Regional Office for South-East Asia (2011) *Addressing Health of the Urban Poor in South-East Asia Region: Challenges and Opportunities.*
3 Wickremasinghe, A.R. and Kasturiratne, A. (2013) *Draft report on Case Studies for Intersectoral Action for health and Health in All Policies in Sri Lanka.* Commissioned by WHO-SEARO (April 2013)

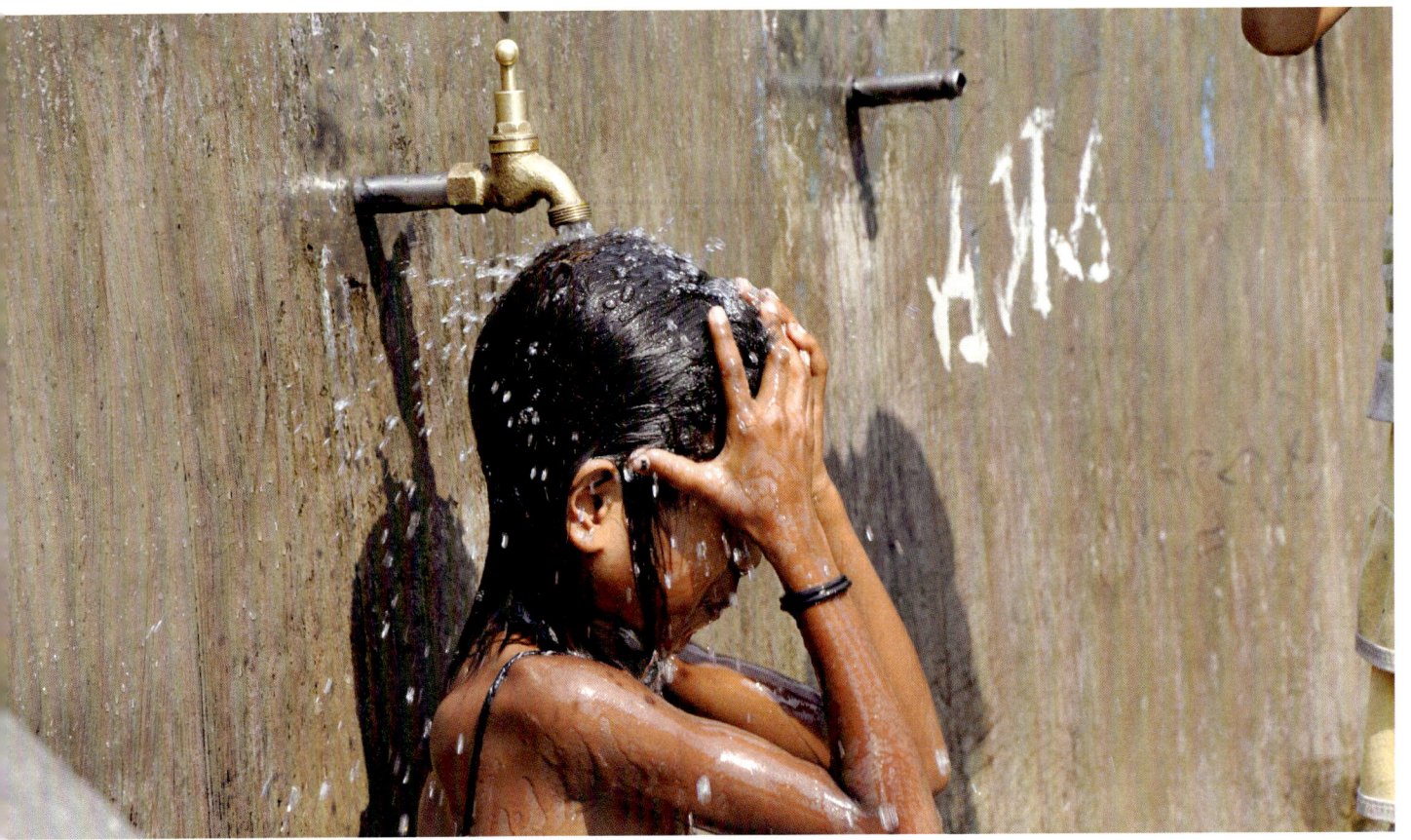
Girl washing in Timor Leste. ©WHO/SEARO/Joao Soares Gusmao

the National Health Security Office are the new mechanisms in Thailand that created synergies across the public sector, business, academia, nongovernmental agencies, and the people. The critical population mass, or assemblie of the people, in Thailand has been seen as an effective way to bring about accountability of the national governance structure (cabinet) through National Health Assemblies, where resolutions are submitted to the cabinet.

5.4 Capacity building

The capacity building that exists in the South-East Asia Region today is very limited. Leadership and support from the legislative framework and political will need to be at the centre for institutional capacity building. However, from the case studies and regional review, only Thailand showed the process of multisectoral engagement of all sectors, people and communities which were empowered. The HIA process in Thailand is an example of where people can demand the assessment using a legislative framework and constitution. Stakeholders, academics, and the National Health Commission play crucial roles in providing support, without a need to establish a conventional institution composed of experts to perform the assessment. The HIA process is one where people's voices and concerns can be heard, though their ability to demand an assessment of an issue or policy, using their rights, as documented in the country's legislative framework and constitution. The HIA model in Thailand is implemented by having people at the centre of actions, to conduct the investigation, assess, collect evidence, and present their health concerns to the authorities involved. The people's capacity was strengthened with synergized support from different groups of academics, stakeholders, and authorities who shared health and public concerns. Through the process, local knowledge and scientific evidence are bridged. Solutions were visualized and sought out in the whole-of-government approach, and also included nongovernmental actors points of views. Public and private solutions to address health impacts of mega-projects and development programmes effecting health were negotiated and agreed upon through a participatory process, so that many countries in South-East Asia began to see the value of Thailand's HIA model and replicate the process.

6. SOUTH-EAST ASIA REGIONAL FRAMEWORK FOR HEALTH IN ALL POLICIES

Building on existing intersectoral/multisectoral actions for health, countries of the WHO South-East Asia Region have developed a framework to strengthen the process towards achieving Health in All Policies. There is agreement that national agendas for Universal Health and reducing health inequity, require a HiAP approach. The regional framework shown here provides the elements of strategic pathways to implement Health in All Policies with appropriate tools and mechanisms to reach common goals and contribute to people's health and equity in the South-East Asia Region.

These are two broad approaches to HiAP that can be considered in the Region:
1. focus on the structural determinants (governance, development policies, equity, human rights, transparency, decentralization, accountability) affecting population health and how they can be addressed at the highest policy levels;
2. focus on intersectoral/multisectoral actions and relevant policies that improve health systems performance (through Universal Health Coverage, Primary Health Care, and other disease control programmes).

A combination could be used in the process to tackle both health systems performance, as well as broader determinants of health, for example, managing NCDs. Many broader determinants of health have an impact on people's health and risk factors for communicable and NCDs. They also have implications for health systems and Universal Health Coverage sustainability. For example, free trade and access to tobacco, which causes lung cancer; poor housing that increases indoor air pollution, causing chronic respiratory disease and an increased risk of tuberculosis; and the absence of a justice system to address human rights violations, which prevent people from having access to social services.

A PHC approach has been prominent in almost all public health interventions in the Region for more than three decades, with a diminished emphasis on broader determinants and social participation as noted. Revitalization of primary health care will strengthen intersectoral/multisectoral actions for health care delivery and health system performance, where people's health can be put at the top of the national agenda, alongside a renewal of multisectoral actions at the policy level. Some countries have already initiated health system reform. The United Nation's dual emphasis on NCDs and Universal Health Coverage will provide an important window of opportunity to put health in other sectors' policies.

However, given complex and diverse sociopolitical conditions within the Region, initiatives could be taken to understand how policies are formulated and when the political climate would be favourable to bring health concerns to policy-makers and provide a window of opportunity in the country context. Instruments/driving forces for Health in All Policies could rely on legislative frameworks, policy options, governance structures, and financial mechanisms.

Universal Health Coverage can be an important entry point to bring the whole government to address health care delivery in a systematic way, rather than only considering health financing. Reduction of health inequity needs to be addressed and responded to through Universal Health Coverage and some of the necessary actions will rely on better governance and using the Health in All Policies approach. Universal Health Coverage aims not only to increase accessibility of health services, but as health is so related to the well-being and prosperity of a nation, it can also partially address socioeconomic causes and consequences of ill health and inequity. It can address issues beyond financing health care costs within the health system. It would do this by using effective intersectoral coordination for prevention services and health promotion as part of overall investments for health.

The whole-of-government approach, as one way of implementing a Health in All Policies approach, can enable the government to address determinants of health and promote health in all levels of public policies, driving other sectors to greater accountability, which would have positive effects on the overall well-being of people and national development.

Universal Health Coverage with a whole-of-government approach could be sustained particularly in low- and medium- income countries, where resources are limited. Joint-financing mechanisms among various public/private sectors with the whole government ensuring universal health coverage, encompassing a preventive, promotive, curative, and rehabilitative approach for all groups of the population would be a way to sustain universal health care. Countries in the Region could benefit from having a whole-of-government approach to prevention of communicable/non-communicable diseases. Promotion of healthy and sustainable environments that support the whole health system should go beyond curative care, where the costs can become increasingly high and unaffordable given competing demands from other sectors like education and security.

Health impact assessment, health lens analysis, and health equity audits/assessment, have been used in varying degrees at different levels of government projects, programmes, activities, with limited influence on policy-makers. In the case of Thailand, the health impact assessment tool was effectively used to raise health concerns from community to parliamentary policy-makers, with a participatory process that drove the health agenda into a number of development policies.

Research to generate evidence of the policy-making process in the Region has been limited or inefficient. Different stages of policy development require different types of evidence in combination with public opinion and political agendas.

A common understanding of health across sectors needs to be advocated with strong evidence to support policy development at different stages. "Healthy people/community/ nation/island" visions that have been developed by different countries in the Region will be a step towards identifying common goals, where shared responsibilities can be identified with concrete outcomes. Intersectoral/multisectoral responses and actions should be relevant to the betterment of the population's health and have policy level influence through advocacy, strategic communication and cross-sectoral dialogues. Applicable tools should be used and assessment should be done on a participatory basis and involve all the relevant sectors, stakeholders and civil societies.

It is recognized that HiAP is an appropriate approach for tackling structural determinants of health, to prevent negative impacts of high-level policies, to measure against emerging epidemics and pandemics of communicable and NCDs, and to address health inequities.

Member States of the South-East Asia Region and partners may consider using the following strategies in moving towards a Health in All Policies approach across public policies.

A. **General strategy at national level** integrates a systemic consideration of health concerns into other sectors' routine policy processes (to promote better quality of life). Integrating health in high-level development goals (such as the post 2015 development agenda) would be a timely opportunity to ensure that health is considered within the whole-of-government approach. Sound public policies across sectors are interrelated to ensure governance structure and financial

Figure 1. Regional framework on Health in All Policies

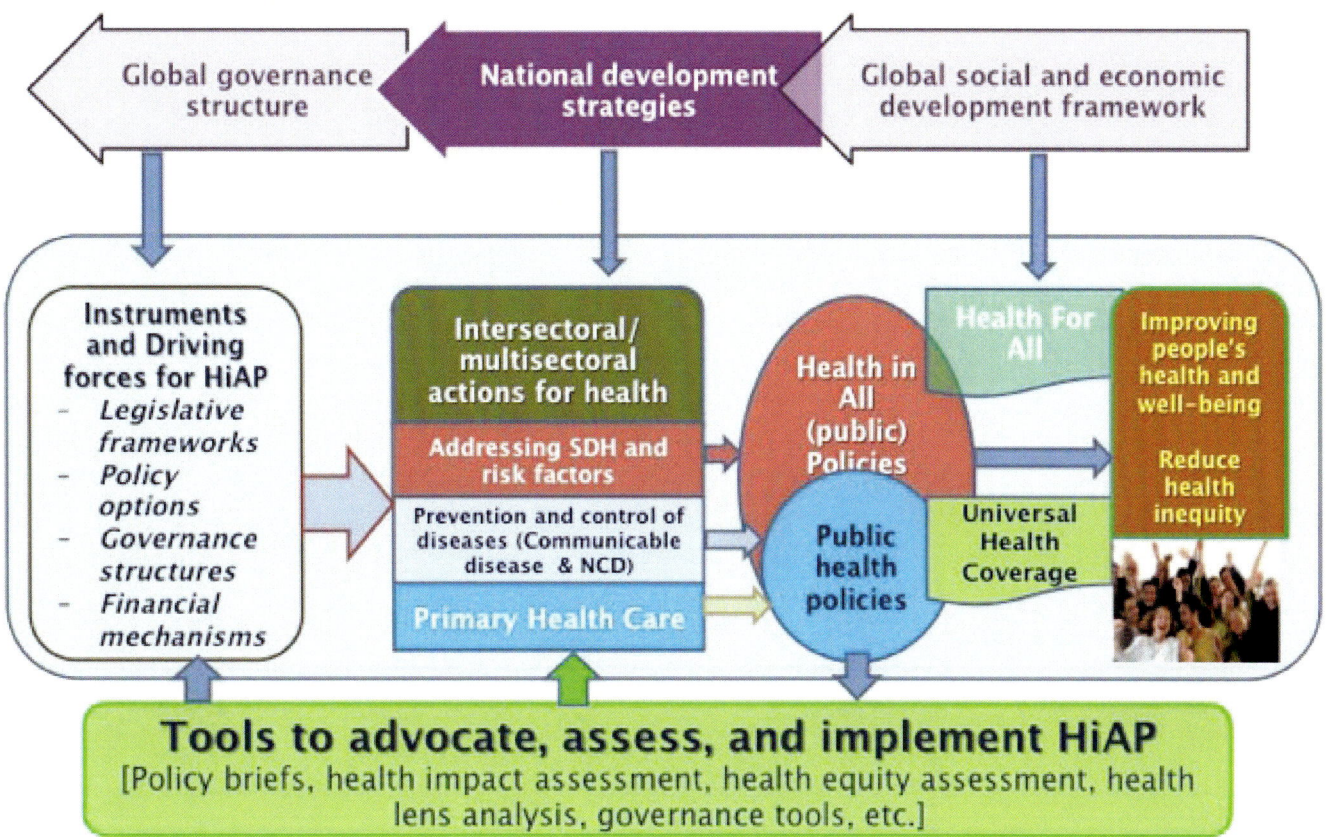

mechanisms that enable public sectors to respond to population health and well-being.

B. **Local/subnational strategy** mediates between general strategic development frameworks and health within the local context to tackle determinants of health in all local policies, such as to address equity and health through promoting health in all urban policies and use health impact assessment and/or health equity tools to engage multisectoral partners.

C. **Issue-centred strategy** integrates specific health concerns into relevant sectors' policies, programmes and activities in disease control and prevention, as well as specific health issues (e.g. WHO FCTC, food security, NCD, road safety, preparation for disaster management).

D. **Combination of the above strategies** as it is applied in a country-specific context can also be initiated. Countries may scale-up their intersectoral/multisectoral programmes on prevention and control throughout national public policies that influence implementation of the programmes, and vice versa[1].

Strong collaborative efforts and incentives across government functions are needed to optimize roles and responsibilities for health and development. What is needed is public-private partnerships and social contracts, NGOs, civil society, academics and the people to support and ensure the reduction of negative impacts of development on health and well-being, to progress towards equity-oriented Universal Health Coverage and accessibility to all social and public services, and to take affirmative actions to promote the health of the population.

---

1 This listing was proposed in the Expert meeting on Health in All Policies, December 2013 held in Bangkok, Thailand and endorsed in the Regional Consultation on Health in All Policies, April 2013 in Colombo, Sri Lanka.

7. WAY FORWARD

Based on the South-East Asian experiences in intersectoral/multisectoral actions, there are many factors/mechanisms/legislations that provide windows of opportunities to enhance the implementation of Health in All Policies to address determinants of health beyond the health sector. These enabling factors include:

› Existing policies engendering the intersectoral process with, e.g. National Commissions, Ministerial Standing Committees, Secretary Level Committees, as well as UN country teams, which could act as effective intersectoral/multisectoral bodies with leadership from high-level government officials. National Social and Economic Development and similar bodies, such as the Gross National Happiness Commission that design and develop national development plans, play a crucial role in ensuring that their development policies and plans do not have negative impacts on health and the livelihoods of the population. The macro-level policy is important to advocate for sound governance structures, coordination, and participation of partners and stakeholders.

› Sectoral policies e.g. human and social security policies, social protection policy, food security, education, poverty reduction policy, transportation, environment, finance, and trade and commerce policies, etc. are key components that link health with other sectors. Health-lens analysis could be a tool for supporting sectoral policies and interventions, and to increase cross-sectoral/intersectoral/multisectoral coordination.

› Decentralized bodies are primary actors which assess the local needs and policy impacts on the people and community at the grass-roots level. Social, economic, environmental, and cultural determinants of health are more immediate at the local level. Decentralization provides opportunities for local governance bodies to directly address health and inequity in their context. However, local capacity needs to be strengthened through a multisectoral participation process, such as the community health impact assessment implemented in Thailand.

› Innovative policy frameworks that bring mutual accountability and shared responsibility, such as comprehensive health and poverty reduction policies with adequate and sustainable financing, transparency, cooperation and coordination; good governance policies for development promoting participations and reoriented delivery systems that ensure sector-wide accountability are required.

› Improving capacity for shared vision, collaborative implementation and policy auditing across sectors ensuring people's physical, mental, social health and well-being are addressed along with each sector's policies and their implementation.

As a result of the Regional Consultation on Health in All Policies in Colombo, Sri Lanka 2013, WHO and Member States are committed to making efforts to implement a Health in All Policies approach, as described in the *South-East Asia Statement for Health in All Policies*, launched and distributed in the 8th Global Conference on Health Promotion in Helsinki, June 2013. These commitments are as follows:

› Raise awareness on Health in All Policies approach within and beyond the health sector.

› Build evidence from broader social determinants of health and policy impacts on health and well-being by countries.

› Build capacity of health promotion practitioners, especially advocacy and leadership skills for policy-level work.

› Develop a National HiAP Plan of Action.

› Utilize existing country intersectoral mechanisms to operationalize HiAP,

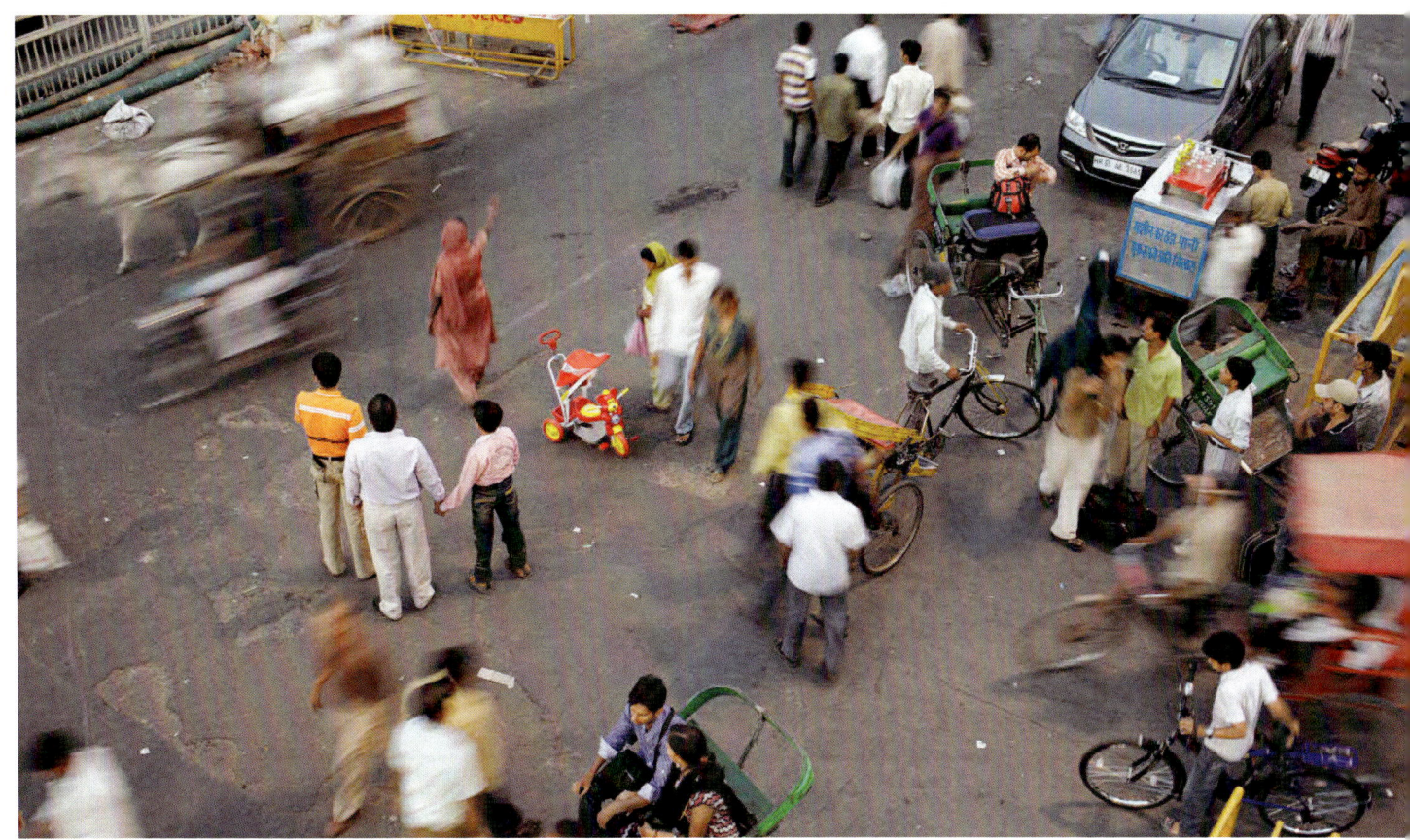

Crowds of evening commuters on a Delhi street, India. ©WHO/Tom Pietrasik

with respect to co-benefits, mutual interests, and conflict of interest among sectors.
- Include health concerns in the policy development process.
- Utilize relevant tools to identify, assess, mobilize, and strengthen multisectoral participation and actions for health.
- Find joint-financial mechanisms to implement HiAP.
- Establish monitoring and assessment for policy-level impacts on health.

Member States have called upon WHO to take following actions:
- WHO at global, regional, and country levels should support capacity building to implement a Health in All Policies approach and provide clear guidance for convincing the health sector on the importance of "health" in all policies, and strengthening collaboration with other sectors.
- WHO should develop a regional database and provide comparative analysis on contributions of interventions addressing inequity and determinants of health across sectors, within and across countries.
- WHO should work together with international partners to provide tools, guidelines, and advocacy materials for strengthening intersectoral/multisectoral actions at policy level particularly on global/regional health priorities such as NCDs, tobacco control, food security, etc.
- WHO, in collaboration with international agencies and partners, should generate evidence for benefits of having Health in All Policies at different levels.
- WHO and international partners should provide channels for policy dialogues and platforms for cross-country/cross-regional sharing of experiences, as well as mobilize joint-financial mechanisms to implement HiAP.
- WHO should coordinate with multisectoral agencies and partners and other UN agencies to lead the health agenda in the Post 2015 Development Goals; WHO should utilize this window of opportunity to mainstream health in all public policies.
- WHO should continue to promote and strengthen healthy settings and scale-up priority settings, such as a healthy cities to advance toward health in all urban policies and/or healthy urban planning.

ANNEX 1:

REGIONAL CASE STUDIES FOR HEALTH IN ALL POLICIES

These case studies were selected through a consultative process with the government agencies and WHO country offices in the Region and through an overall review of the regional situation on intersectoral actions for social determinants of health. WHO Regional Office for South-East Asia facilitated a series of discussions with governmental counterparts and technical units. Inventory of the past decade of experiences in technical units and regional reports in libraries was used to guide regional development for the framework and in-depth country case studies. An intersectoral action analytic framework has been used to investigate the particularities of each case. Some of the cases did not have earlier documentation and have been left out of WHO records. Substitute procedures, such as stakeholders meetings and consultations with policy-makers in countries were used to bring out country best experiences.

Themes from the 8th Global Conference on Health Promotion (Helsinki) Addressed						
In-depth case study topic	Global policy-making	Political will and processes	Health promotion, health equity (and Primary Health Care)	Economics	Social change	Capacity building
Implementing Tobacco Control Policy and Gross National Happiness audits in Bhutan: existing, vital mechanisms for Health in All Policies *(1)*	●	●	●			
Happiness for health and health for happiness. Determinants of health in the context of Gross National Happiness in Bhutan.		●				
Identifying common responsibilities for tobacco control: the WHO Framework Convention for Tobacco Control in India	●	●			●	
Nutrition and nutrition-sensitive interventions as an opportunity for institutionalizing Health in All Policies: the Multisectoral Nutrition Programme in Nepal *(1)*		●	●			
Learning from local cases and innovation to address the social determinants of health in Sri Lanka: the Metro Colombo Urban Development Project *(1,3)*			●	●		
Learning from local cases and innovation to address the social determinants of health in Sri Lanka: the Alawwa Health Project*(1,3,4)*			●		●	●
Thailand's National Health Assembly: People's Power for Health in All Policies Approach		●	●		●	●
Strategic development plans as important entry points for a Health in All Policies approach: the case of Timor-Leste post-conflict *(1)*		●			●	

(1) Funded by WHO Ethics and Social Determinants of Health Department through Rockefeller Foundation grant for, Supporting Regional Positions on Health in All Policies, with WHO SEARO and WHO country offices for Bhutan, Nepal, Sri Lanka, and Timor-Leste
(2) Funded by WHO Kobe Centre in collaboration with WHO SEARO and WHO Country Offices for India and Thailand
(3) Funded by WHO Ethics and Social Determinants of Health Department through the Lighthouse Project, supported by a specified grant from the Government of Brazil

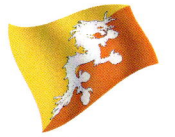

Bhutan

Implementing Tobacco Control Policy and Gross National Happiness policy serving in Bhutan: existing, vital mechanisms for Health in All Policies[1]

The Bhutanese people believe that good health brings happiness and well-being, thus underlining health as one of the determinants of happiness. The Royal Government of Bhutan accords a high priority to the promotion of health and happiness of its population through the model of Gross National Happiness (GNH). The government integrates the GNH values into all of the national policy-making processes. Health is one of the core domains of GNH and is part and parcel of the policy screening process.

The concept of "Health in All Policies" (HiAP) is fairly new to the Bhutanese policy-makers and planners, including those in the Ministry of Health. However, a multisectoral approach, implemented through intergovernmental and multisectoral committees or task forces platforms, involving actors from civil society, consumer groups and academia, is a mechanism that has been used. Using this platform means the health sector can seek support from other sectors, and make necessary decisions in the process of policy development. The Tobacco Control Board is an example. It was created in Bhutan, where a Board comprises 13 members representing different governmental and other agencies.

The context of this case is the increasing political will that emerged in Bhutan to improve tobacco control. The Ministry of Health has played a leading role since the 1980s in providing information to the public and other sectors to reduce and control tobacco use. However, when the multisectoral committee was established in the 1990s at the national and district levels, other sectors were invited to support better cooperation and interactions with the Ministry of Health. Subsequently, in 2004 and 2005, the sale of tobacco was banned and smoke-free areas designated, the success of which was invariably attributed to intersectoral efforts, rather than health alone. The Tobacco Control Act of Bhutan was brought in, in 2010. It played a crucial role in empowering the enforcement and response of agencies, enabling them to carry out their responsibilities without fear or ambiguity. Intersectoral actions are evident in the enforcement of tobacco control policy, whereby the measures of reducing tobacco use in the country are integrated into the plans of other sectors. Community leaders and district officers also play a crucial role in monitoring tobacco control measures. This range of intersectoral actions may have contributed positively towards reducing tobacco consumption and maintaining low prevalence rates of tobacco use in Bhutan, thereby effectively helping with compliance with the provisions of the WHO FCTC. The case study clearly demonstrated the feasibility of using intersectoral mechanisms in policy development and the gains from improving the efficiency of cooperation and coordination between sectors.

In recent years, the Royal Government of Bhutan approved a number of new public policies which took health concerns into consideration. The GNH Commission is responsible for processing all the policy proposals for approval using the "GNH policy screening tool" to check or "audit" all policies for their negative implications on health and inconsistency with the other GNH indicators. The policies can then be recommended for revision or rejection.

Currently, policy-makers are of the view that it would be wise to use these existing mechanisms as entry points to introduce HiAP. With this strategic approach in mind, Gross National Happiness Commission and the Ministry of Health need to work out an appropriate modality for the initiation of an HiAP approach, and eventually to achieve the goals of HiAP for the country.

---

1 Prepared by Sonam Rinchen, Former Temporary International Professional, WHO Tobacco Free Initiative, Regional Office for South-East Asia, and currently freelance academic in Bhutan. This summary is an abridged version from a longer case study (see Rinchen S, 2013).

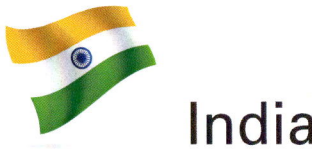

India

Identifying common responsibilities for tobacco control: the WHO Framework Convention for Tobacco Control in India[2]

The estimated number of adult tobacco users in India is 274.9 million, with 206 million users of only smokeless tobacco. Prevalence of overall tobacco use among males is 48% and that among females is 20%. The myriad of ways in which tobacco is produced, marketed and consumed further adds to the complexities of tobacco control. This case study describes how intersectoral actions for health have contributed to the implementation of the WHO Framework Convention on Tobacco Control (WHO FCTC) in India and thereby offers insights for Health in All Policies.

The WHO FCTC, ratified by the Government of India in 2004, provides the foundation to manage tobacco control programmes and requires the cooperation of related sectors. A high-level governance structure, the National Tobacco Control Cell, was established in the Ministry of Health and Family Welfare in collaboration with WHO Country Office for India for overall policy formulation, planning, monitoring and evaluation of the different activities envisaged under the programme. Every State has a State Tobacco Control Cell that is responsible for planning, implementation and monitoring at State level. To drive the implementation of the WHO FCTC by different sectors, high-level coordination committees have been established at national, state and district levels.

The ministries that have contributed towards tobacco control at national and state level include: Ministry of Human Resource Development, Ministry of Information and Broadcasting, Ministry of Home Affairs, Ministry of Labour, Ministry of Railways and Ministry of Finance. In addition Parliament, the judiciary, civil society and media have also been significant allies for the advancement of tobacco control in India. Preliminary work is underway with the Ministry of Agriculture, Ministry of Labour, Department of Rural Development and Ministry of Environment and Forest for working out strategies to provide alternative livelihoods for those engaged in rolling cigarettes, harvesting and tobacco cultivation.

The intersectoral experience of the tobacco control programme found some challenges to be addressed, such as like low levels of involvement of other ministries and the perception that "tobacco control is the mandate of the Ministry of Health alone". They are being addressed through advancing mechanisms for advocacy and dialogue with stakeholders, including training. Sensitization and training workshops on key topics are held regularly to help multisectoral stakeholders/ministries understand their roles and how to implement the provisions of WHO FCTC. Detailed guidelines have been developed to further help all programme implementers and law enforcers, regardless of sector or level of government.

Through the various processes described above, India has been able to achieve varying levels of compliance on most of the key provisions of WHO FCTC and MPOWER package. New policy initiatives have come into force on the prohibition of the sale of tobacco to minors and around educational institutions, imposing restrictions on tobacco imagery in films and TV programmes and a ban on smokeless tobacco products like 'gutka' (chewed tobacco). Some states, cities and villages have come forward and declared their jurisdictions as smoke-free and tobacco-free. The continued roll out of and enforcement of these new initiatives will continue to rely on cooperation and collaboration across sectors, as well as the different levels of government, supported by appropriate advocacy and training.

---

[2] Prepared by Anushree Mishra. This summary is an abridged version from a case study that is also published as a stand-alone publication by the WHO Country Office of India.

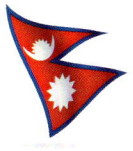

Nepal

Nutrition and nutrition-sensitive interventions as an opportunity for institutionalizing Health in All Policies: the Multisectoral Nutrition Programme in Nepal[3]

The case study examines the work of the Multisectoral Nutrition Programme, established in Nepal in 2012. This programme was established following a recognized string of multisectoral nutrition initiatives in Nepal that have been going since the 1970s. Integrated Rural Development (IRD) projects, such as Rasuwa Nuwakot IRD and Mahakali IRD in the 1970s, built on a holistic approach to development that attempted to address multiple constraints simultaneously through appropriate planning for development priorities. Development areas of focus included health and nutrition, agriculture, education, and rural roads. A nutrition coordination committee was established as a result of these processes in the National Planning Commission in 1977. In the 1980's the Nepal Joint Nutrition Support Programme (JNSP) was initiated (in 1985) by WHO and UNICEF with the support of the Italian government. However, the JNSP was not continued because of inadequate capacity, a lack of health infrastructure at village level, fluctuating donor policies and support among many other reasons.

In 2012, the Multisectoral Nutrition Programme was initiated, which focused on specific interventions, such as improving feeding, care practices in the health sector, and nutrition-sensitive interventions for families and communities. Nutrition-sensitive interventions are comprised of interventions led by other sectors, including those aimed at addressing food availability, affordability, access, and quality of food. A multisectoral planning framework was used to define strategic objectives, interventions, expected outputs, estimated budget, and monitoring indicators for each sector. The planning framework, coupled with existing decentralized governance structure under the mandate of the Local Self Governance Act (1999), included expansion of infrastructure for public health, education, and agriculture. With multiple sectors involved, and a broad concept of health interventions that include nutrition-sensitive interventions, the Multisectoral Nutrition Programme provides a current window of opportunity for institutionalization of Health in All Policies in Nepal.

---

[3] Prepared by Dr Suniti Acharya, Executive Director, Centre for Health Policy Research and Dialogue (CHPRD), Kathmandu, Nepal. This summary is an abridged version from a longer case study that is currently being finalized for publication.

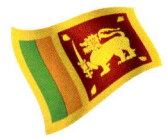

Sri Lanka

Learning from local cases and innovation to address the social determinants of health in Sri Lanka: the Metro Colombo Urban Development Project and the Alawwa Health Project[4]

Sri Lanka has a long history of public health legislation dating back to the colonial era. The first such legislature titled "Nuisances Ordinance No 15 of 1862" focused on better preservation of public health and the suppression of nuisances. For the time, it was essentially a piece of legislature that focused on intersectoral collaboration. The 1970s and 1980s witnessed the "good health at low cost" case studies – one of which focused on Sri Lanka. Sri Lanka's efforts to simultaneously champion universal provision of education and health – seemingly, tied to a common vision of development – were examples also cited at the launch of the WHO Commission on Social Determinants and Health. Following the end of the WHO Commission on Social Determinants of Health in 2008, Sri Lanka continued to search for innovative ways to put WHO recommendations into practice to address the social determinants of health. One of the two case studies therefore focuses on an innovative pilot project addressing the social determinants of health through primary health care and citizen's participation. The other case focuses on how a recent instance of an intersectoral natural disaster prevention and infrastructure development project, that excluded local health authorities, can nevertheless boost health outcomes. It then offers insights into the rationale for engaging the health sector. Both cases provide insights into how the local level can be an entry point for applying Health in All Policies approaches.

In the case of the **Metro-Colombo Urban Development Project**, The Ministry of Defence and Urban Development is in charge of the project to reduce flood risks and to improve urban infrastructure and services with financial assistance from the World Bank. The project consists of two components. The first component focuses on interventions to address the urgent issue of urban flooding, which regularly paralyzes the economy of the Colombo Metropolitan Area with high socio-economic costs. This component finances both structural and non-structural activities related to flood control and drainage management identified as a priority by the interagency Flood Mitigation Task Force. Its implementation requires social and environmental impact assessments, in particular for more complicated interventions with substantial changes to drainage systems and water transportation within the city. The second component focuses on urban development and infrastructure rehabilitation for Metro Colombo Local Authorities through (a) strengthening strategic planning processes at the metropolitan level and (b) supporting local authorities to: (i) rehabilitating and managing their drainage infrastructure and streets; and (ii) improving solid waste collection.

The key social risks and issues identified in the social impact assessment related to this second component were (i) mitigating potential involuntary resettlement and any adverse impacts on physical and cultural resources; (ii) promoting social inclusion and accountability; and (iii) supporting sustainable management for resettlement sites developed. While an interview of the Chief Medical Officer of Health of the Colombo Municipal Council indicated that neither he nor the Public Health Department of the Colombo Municipal Council were involved in the planning, implementation, or the monitoring and evaluation of the project thus far, positive results have been observed for health. These include lower pollution levels, reduction of dengue fever incidence that had been prevalent in the areas with slum dwellings.

---

[4] Prepared by Professor A.R. Wickremasinghe and Dr Anuradhani Kasturiratne, Department of Public Health, Faculty of Medicine, University of Kelaniya, Sri Lanka. This summary is an abridged version from a longer case study that is currently being finalized for publication.

The following facts are highlighted with regard to lessons for the implementation of a Health in All Policies approach.

- Although the health sector may not have been formally consulted within the design and implementation of this project, the "health" aspect was considered by others. This may be true of other projects and policies occurring elsewhere. The health sector should consider why and when similar developments may be occurring without explicit consideration of health, and when their involvement is necessary and useful.
- An assessment of the social impact assessment study revealed that it is possible that the involvement of the health sector would have improved the interventions introduced in the project, especially when considering alternate residential facilities. Allocating residents formerly living in informal dwellings to high-rise constructions has health risks. The effective size, in view of the high-rise nature of the accommodation and the larger average family size of the resettled occupants may not be optimal for the future health prospects of these residents. Providing psychosocial support to affected persons in the implementation of the project may have also been an important contribution.

The Alawwa Health Project was initiated in the Alawwa Divisional Secretariat area of the Kurunegala District of the North Western Province of Sri Lanka to address health inequalities through coordinated actions on social determinants of health and revitalization of the Primary Health Care approach. The Alawwa Divisional Secretariat area of the Kurunegala District of the North Western Province of Sri Lanka has a population of approximately 63 889 spread over an area of 70 km^2. It is a rural area with an economy based primarily on agriculture predominantly with paddy and coconut cultivation. Alawwa Divisional Secretariat comprises mostly traditional villages where generations of families have lived in the area for long periods of time. There is some form of a caste system operating in the villages with their own traditions being passed down within generations. Most of the older persons are not that well educated, with the majority educated up to grade 8 or 10. According to the medical officer of health of the area, the main health problems were dengue fever and, in the past, leptospirosis. The officer also reiterated that poverty is a major problem in the area, with every third person owning lands that have been neglected, thereby contributing to the dengue fever problem. There is a relatively good transport system. A large number of people work in garment factories. Based on the distribution of health care institutions, health care is available to most persons within four kilometres.

Specific aims of the project were to introduce a Health in All Policies centred on the Primary Health Care model, to reduce and mitigate the inequalities caused by social determinants of health. A number of activities were undertaken to contribute to these objectives. Interim reports, interviews and focus groups with project implementers indicate that the project has achieved some noteworthy results. In particular the experiences of Health Promotion Villages have been successful. The concept of a health promotion village was based on the perceived needs of villagers to tackle common problems such as poor nutrition practices, alcohol abuse and controlling NCDs. Initially, 15 consenting villagers from each village are requested to attend an initial meeting with the public health midwife of the area, the field worker who is primarily in charge of maternal and child health, to form a committee that would liaise on health promotion activities in the village. Other villagers are also invited to join at any time, if they so wish. This group then identifies problems they perceive as important. The problems are analysed and suitable solutions are worked out considering the resources available and the advice of the medical officer of health. The programme was initially started in 12 villages in 8 areas with public health midwifes but seeing the results of the project, the demand has increased from other villages.

Overall, this work has yielded several insights for Health in All Policies from the Primary Health Care and local levels. These include:

> It is easy to get other sectors involved in health-related projects through the Primary Health Care approach. The Primary Health Care Approach is closely engaged with the community at grass-roots level. Trust between sectors had to be established but this is more easily done at grass-roots level. The community created the demand for services that would benefit them as individuals and as a community. This required empowerment of the community. Community demand for consideration of Health in All Policies may be a better option for an entry point for the institutionalization of the Health in All Policies approach, as opposed to a top-down approach. This may also be used to sensitize policy-makers on the need for, and the benefits of, considering "Health" in All Policies. Here "policies" were taken to refer to decisions on the distribution of resources and services taken at the local government and district level.

> The experience of the project participants was that working with local government authorities required less time on coordination activities. Their commitment was also evident in terms of an annual budget allocation of 23% for health-related activities.

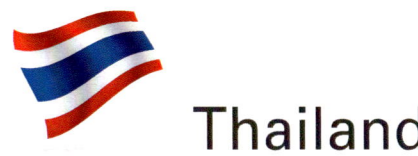

Thailand

Thailand's National Health Assembly: "people's power for a Health in All Policies approach"[5]

A broader definition of "health" has traditionally been applied in the health sector and across government in Thailand, recognizing that health is influenced by a number of determinants inside and outside the health sector. Thus, the concept of "Health in All Policies" was gradually introduced. In 2000, the National Health System Reform Committee and the National Health System Reform Office were established to steer the health systems reform in Thailand and mandated to draft the National Health Bill that was discussed, revised and completed with more than 500 brainstorming sessions participated by over 400 000 people from various sectors and organizations. The National Health Act 2007 involved a radical paradigm shift in the health system, which includes physical, mental, spiritual and social aspects interrelated holistically in a balanced manner. The Act serves as an effective legal framework to set guidelines on the national health development in which all parties in society, not only the health sector, have a stake through participatory approaches and intersectoral actions. The broader scope of health and the emphasis on the importance of the participatory process have led to the establishment of a new organization structure, the National Health Commission, chaired by the Prime Minister, consisting of three major constituencies: (1) the government sector, (2) the professional sector, and (3) the people sector.

According to the National Health Act (2007), "health assembly" is defined as a process in which the public and related government agencies exchange their knowledge and cordially learn from each other through an organizing systematic forum with public participation, leading to suggestion of healthy public policies to improve the health of populations. The health assembly can be organized at different levels (local-based, area-based, and national health assemblies). The National Health Assembly (NHA) was established to serve as a public space for active engagement by all sectors and stakeholders including civil society. The NHA process is radically different from a conventional policy-making one, where government and academic sectors are the sole powers with its top-down nature. In contrast, the NHA process generates a "soft power" and provides a "social space" for civil society to have active participation in policy engagement. It increasingly brings all partners from the three powers on board and deliberations are increasingly based on evidence.

All of the NHA resolutions are submitted to the Cabinet, for either acknowledgment or approval for further actions by concerned departments, ministries and agencies. The National Health Commission also established the Monitoring and Evaluation Committee as a mechanism to continuously follow the progress and impacts of the resolutions. One of the lessons learned was that although the adopted resolutions have passed through the Cabinet and become public policies, responsible agencies mandated in the resolutions need to be active enough to translate policies into practice through intersectoral actions. From the past NHAs, each resolution has different characteristics in intersectoral movement. Intersectoral works between health and non-health sectors remain fragmented, especially in response to the mitigation of health impacts generated by government policies. Challenges in bringing intersectoral responses include: trust building among constituencies, conflict of interests of different sectors, inadequate knowledge or evidence, and inadequate understanding of the participatory process of the NHA and concept of Health in All Policies.

---

5   Prepared by Tipicha Posayanonda, Nattaya Thaennin, Orapan Srisookwatana, The National Health Commission Office, Nonthaburi, Thailand. This summary is an abridged version from a longer case study that is currently being finalized for publication.

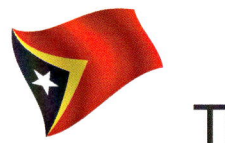

Timor-Leste

Strategic development plans as important entry points for a Health in All Policies approach: the case of Timor-Leste post-conflict[6]

Timor-Leste does not have an explicit Health in All Policies approach that it has applied. Yet the intent for intersectoral actions for health has been expressed in national and health policy documents. To date, as elsewhere, the implementation has been mixed. Any important legislation or project has to be approved by the Presidency of Council of Ministers that consists of the Prime Minister, the Vice Prime Minister and the ministers. However, the cross-disciplinary nature of this exercise is not reflected in the implementation.

Timor-Leste is classified as a fragile state. As such, it has established a plan for transition from a phase of internal security to the next development phase of state building (Transition Plan 2011). The objective of rebuilding the State is on its way. Much of Timor-Leste's health infrastructure was destroyed during the independence struggle and has since been rebuilt. Timor-Leste's public health system is decentralized.

The country has now established systems of national governance. Timor-Leste successfully completed presidential and parliamentary elections in 2002, 2006, 2007 and 2012. The United Nations Integrated Mission in Timor-Leste came to an end on 31 December 2012. The country is still in the process of formulating policies and legislation. The Timor-Leste Strategic Development Plan 2011–2030 was launched in July 2011. It provides a long-term development vision and covers three key areas: social capital, infrastructure development and economic development. Social capital includes education and training, health, social inclusion, environment, culture and heritage. It builds on the 2002 National Development Plan and 'Timor-Leste – A Vision for 2020'. Over 70 community consultations in "sucos" (villages) across Timor-Leste were part of the Strategic Development Plan development process.

In the formulation of policies as part of the Strategic Development Plan, the health sector has collaborated with education, social services, agriculture, infrastructure, state administration, transportation and police. However, engagement with the finance sector has been limited to the budgetary process. Experience thus far indicates that intersectoral work has been hampered by a lack of financial and human resources, and limited inter/intrasectoral coordination capacity within the health ministry, which includes a limited understanding of where the substantive interlinkage among sectors is. Despite these challenges there are facilitating factors for intersectoral actions for health. These include the opportunities afforded by the overall strategic framework, as well as the vision of health prevailing within the health sector as exemplified by the Intersectoral Action Framework for well-being and health (a framework for action) that was formulated in 2005 as an inter-ministerial strategy, using an integrated primary health care approach. The strategy identifies the key diseases in Timor-Leste and links with 'key determinants' (social determinants) of health. It proposed an Intersectoral Action Framework which provides direction for joint government and community action, but its status as a policy tool is not yet certain. Its key components may yet offer insights into how health can address the issue of interlinkages with other policy sectors.

They include:
> Reduction in negative environmental determinants of health and well-being (water, air, sanitation, food supply and quality, physical safety, etc.);
> Treatment of illness, prevention initiatives and interventions for common disabilities;
> Improving knowledge, skills and competencies for individuals and groups;
> Enabling better use of and improving access to essential resources to those in need;
> Strengthening social support mechanisms, practices and policies.

---

[6] Prepared by Dr Shilpa Pandav, Health Economist, International consultant, Timor-Leste. This summary is an abridged version from a longer case study that is currently being finalized for publication.

ANNEX 2:
SOUTH-EAST ASIA REGION STATEMENT ON HEALTH IN ALL POLICIES

SOUTH-EAST ASIA REGION
HiAP Statement

Message from the Regional Director

Outcome of the Regional Consultation on HiAP, April 2013

After several movements focusing on "health promotion" and "social determinants of health", the idea of health in all policies (HiAP) is rapidly gaining global attention. It is also being recognized that multisectoral and multidisciplinary actions to tackle new challenges such as noncommunicable diseases, climate changes, food security, urbanization and health, are essential. To address these challenges, multisectoral partnerships are needed and, several sectors need to work together as equal partners to achieve positive outcomes that are mutually beneficial.

The regional framework includes:

1. Recognition of broader determinants of health
2. Strategic directions for implementation
3. Tools and mechanisms
4. Roles of health sector
5. Roles of non-health sectors
6. Monitoring progress

Our commitment towards the "health for all" goal could be renewed and strengthened through a more operational approach to implement health in all policies at all levels. Political commitment at the highest levels will ensure that the vision of "health for all" and "all for health" is realized soon through efficient and coordinated implementation of various initiatives by all sectors.

We are progressing towards achieving the Millennium Development Goals (MDG) and are positioning ourselves for post-2015 development. We need to take this opportunity to reaffirm and strengthen our multisectoral efforts to ensure health is at the centre of the development agenda and encourage other sectors to realize the impacts their policies may have on the population's well-being.

When we move towards the attainment of health for all through universal health coverage, effective involvement of other sectors through the "HiAP" approach becomes more necessary to ensure affordable and sustainable national health development. We may also keep in mind that, with "strategic considerations" and "focused actions" exerted under strong policy back up at the highest level we will be able to work successfully for people's health through "HiAP".

Dr Samlee Plianbangchang

The Common mission for "health" goes beyond the health sector because underlying causes of ill-health are determined by actions and impacts of policies from other sectors.

Regional Framework on HiAP

Building on existing intersectoral/multisectoral actions for health, countries of the WHO South-East Asia Region have developed a framework to strengthen the process towards achieving health in all policies. There is agreement that national agendas for universal health coverage, improving people's health and reducing health inequity require a HiAP approach. The regional framework provides strategic pathways to implement health in all policies with appropriate tools and mechanisms to reach common goals and contribute to people's health and equity in South-East Asia.

The framework provides options for strategic directions. Based on their specific context, countries, including governance structures and mechanisms, may adopt a general overarching strategy for HiAP at the national level or adopt local/subnational strategies. An alternative could be issue-centred strategies involving health and one or more relevant sector(s) to tackle a specific issue. Countries can also adopt a combination of strategies for implementation. Tools such as health impact assessment-HIA, health-lens analysis, and governance tool could be used to engage other sectors to address underlying issues affecting health. Existing mechanisms in countries such as national development commissions and UNDAF were recommended to be important mechanisms to draw multisectoral actions for health.

Commitments

Drawing from the Adelaide Statement on Health in All Policies 2010, Member States recognize that health in all policies is a new social contract between all sectors to advance human development, to ensure sustainability and equity; and to improve health outcomes. This requires engagement of leaders and policy makers at all levels of government – local, regional, and international.

It is recognized that HiAP is an appropriate approach to tackle structural determinants of health, to prevent negative impacts of high-level policies, to measure against emerging epidemics and pandemics of communicable and noncommunicable diseases, and to address health inequity.

Strong collaborative efforts across government functions are needed to optimize roles and responsibilities for health and development of the people. What is needed is public-private partnerships, nongovernmental agencies, civil society, academics and the people to support and ensure reduction of negative impacts of development on health and well-being, to ensure universal coverage and accessibility to health and social services, and to take affirmative actions to improve the health of the population.

The government plays crucial roles in ensuring intersectoral/ multisectoral coordination for health at the highest level.

Framework on HiAP for South-East Asia

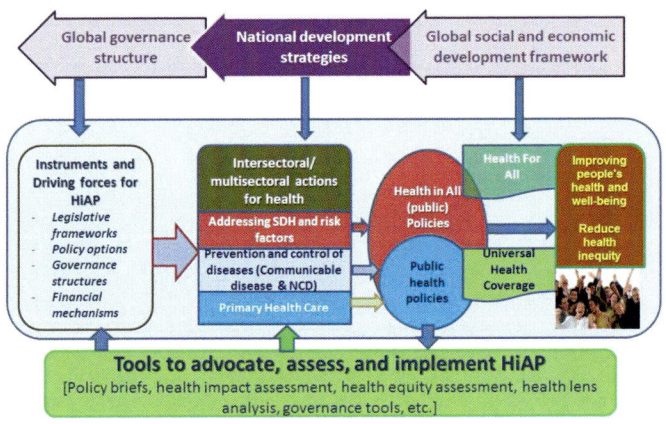

WAY FORWARD

- Raise awareness on health in all policies approach within and beyond health sector.
- Build evidence from broader social determinants of health and policy impacts on health and well-being by countries.
- Build capacity of health promotion practitioners, especially advocacy and leadership skills for policy-level work.
- Develop National HiAP Plan of Action.
- Utilize existing country intersectoral mechanisms to operationalize HiAP, with respect to co-benefits, mutual interests, and conflict of interest among sectors.
- Include health concerns in the policy development process.
- Utilize relevant tools to identify, assess, mobilize, and strengthen multisectoral participation and actions for health.
- Find joint-financial mechanism to implement HiAP.
- Establish monitoring and assessment for policy level impacts on health.

Contact

Dr Suvajee Good, Programme Coordinator,
Health promotion & social determinants of health
Department of Sustainable Development and Healthy Environment
WHO Regional Office for South-East Asia
9 IP Estate, Mahatma Gandhi Marg
New Delhi, India 110002
E-mail: goods@who.int

BIBLIOGRAPHY

Attanayake N (2001). *An assessment of the effectiveness of decentralization of health services in Sri Lanka.* In, Qadeer I, Sen K and Nayar KR, eds. (2001). Public health and the poverty of reforms: The South Asian Predicament. New Delhi: Sage. pp. 398-412.

Bhattacharya S (2010). *The World Health Organization and the Social Determinants of Health: Assessing Theory, Policy and Practice.* Social Determinants of Health Assessing Theory, Policy and Practice

Buasai S, Kanchanachitra C, Siwaraksa P (2007). The way forward: experiences of health promotion development in Thailand. *Promotion & Education* 14 (4): 250-253.

Buckett K (2010). "Editorial", Public Health Bulletin SA, Health in All Policies, *Adelaide 2010 International Meeting Volume 7 (Number 2).*

Chuengsatiansup K (2008). *Deliberative Action: Civil Society and Health Systems Reform in Thailand.* Nonthaburi: National Health Commission Office.

Fernando DF (2001). *Structural Adjustment Programs and Health Care services in Sri Lanka: an overview.* In, Qadeer I, Sen K and Nayar KR, eds. (2001). Public health and the poverty of reforms: The South Asian Predicament. New Delhi: Sage. pp. 311-326.

Fotso JC, Friel S, Khadr Z, Meresman S, Patil-Deshmukh A, Saenz R, Salgado N (2010). *Social Conditions and Urban Health Inequities.* Working Paper Global Research Network on Urban Health Equity.

Friel S and Baker PI (2009). *Equity, food security and health equity in the Asia Pacific region.* Asia Pac J Clin Nutr 2009;18(4):620-632.

Gunatilleke, G (1984) Ed. *Intersectoral linkages and health development: Case studies in India (Kerala State), Jamaica, Norway, Sri Lanka and Thailand.* WHO Offset Publication No.83, Geneva: World Health Organization.

Gunatilleke, G (2007). *Inter-sectoral Action for Health the Sri Lankan Case Study.* The Marga Institute.

Hadi A (2001). Promoting health knowledge through micro credit programmes: experiences of BRAC in Bangladesh. *Health promotion International*, 16(3):219-227.

ICSSR-ICMR. *Health for all: An alternative strategy.* Pune: Indian Institute of Education; 1981

Kickbusch, I (2010). *Health in All Policies: the evolution of the concept of horizontal health governance.* Implementing Health in All Policies: Adelaide 2010. I. Kickbusch and K. Buckett. Adelaide, Department of Health, Government of South Australia: 11–23.

Krech R (2010). *Reflections on the Adelaide 2010 Health in All Policies International Meeting.* Public Health Bulletin SA, Health in All Policies, Adelaide 2010 International Meeting Volume 7, (No. 2).

Ministry of Public Health (2007). *School Health Program in Thailand:* Case study Presented to World Health Organization by School age and Youth Health Group, Bureau of Health Promotion, Department of Health, Thailand, December 2007.

Mukhopadhyay A (2007). South Asia's health promotion kaleidoscope. *Promotion & Education, 2007*, XIV (4): pp 238-243

Mulgan G (2010). *Holistic government and what works.* Public Health Bulletin SA, Health in All Policies, Adelaide 2010 International Meeting Volume 7(No. 2).

Murray CJL and Lopez AD (2004). Monitoring global health: time for new solutions. *BMJ* ;329:1096

Mushtaque A, Chowdhury R, Bhuiya A (2001). *Do poverty alleviation programmes reduce inequities in health? The Bangladesh experience. In Poverty, Inequality and Health: An International Perspective* Edited by: Leon DA, Walt G. Oxford: Oxford University Press; 313-331Mannheimer, L. N., J. Lehto, et al. (2007). "Window of opportunity for intersectoral health policy in Sweden—open, half-open or half-shut?" *Health Promotion International,* Vol. 22(No. 4).

National Health Commission Office (2010). *National Health Act, Thailand 2007.* Nonthaburi: National Health Commission Office.

National Health Commission Office (2010). *Thailand's rules and Procedures for the Health Impact Assessment of Public Policies.* Nonthaburi: Health Impact Assessment Coordinating Unit, NHCO

Nayar KR (1998). Old priorities and new agenda of public health in India: is there a mismatch? *Croat. Med J;* 39 (3): 308-315

Nayar KR (2001). *Politics of Decentralization: Lessons from Kerala.* In, Qadeer I, Sen K and Nayar KR, eds. (2001). Public health and the poverty of reforms: The South Asian Predicament. New Delhi: Sage. pp. 363-378.

Nayar KR (2007). Social exclusion, caste and health: A review based on the social determinants framework. *Indian J Med Res,* 126: 355-363

Pandav SM (2012). *(Draft) Documentation on implementation of Health in All Policies in the South-East Asia Region.* September, 2012. New Delhi: WHO-SEARO

Patcharanarumol W et al., (2011). *Why and how did Thailand achieve good health at low cost?* London: LSHTM.

Pengkam S (2012). *12 years of HIA in Thailand.* Presentation made at Meeting of Experts on Measuring Health Equity and Health Impact Assessment towards Health in All Policies WHO/SEARO, New Delhi 6-8 June 2012.

Perera, M A L R (2006). *Intersectoral Action for Health in Sri Lanka.* A case study commissioned by the Health Systems Knowledge Network.

PHFI. *High Level Expert Group Report on Universal Health Coverage for India.* Instituted by Planning Commission. New Delhi: PHFI; 2011.

Posayanonda T, Thaennin N and Srisookwatana O (undated). *Thailand's National Health Assembly: Intersectoral action for health.* Nonthaburi: The National Health Commission Office.

Puska P, Stahl T (2010). "Health in All Policies – The Finnish initiative: background, principles and current issues." *Annual Review of Public Health,* 31: 315-328.

Rinchen S (2013) Case Study on *Implementation of Tobacco Control Policy in Bhutan: A Vital Platform for Intersectoral Actions,* commissioned by WHO-SEARO, March 2013.

Royal Government of Bhutan (2011). *Royal Government of Bhutan Decade of Action for Road Safety (2011-2020)*

Royal Government of Bhutan Commitment to the Decade of Action for Road Safety (2011–2020).

Sachs J (2012). Introduction. In, Helliwell J, Layard R and Sachs J eds. *World Happiness Report.*

SEWA (2000). *Promoting health security for women in the informal sector.* Ahmedabad: Self Employed Women's Association

Silva K T (2010). *Social Determinants of Health: Lessons from Sri Lanka. Social Determinants of Health Assessing Theory, Policy and Practice.* S. Bhattachrya, S. Messenger and C. Overy, Orient Blackswan Private Limited.

Ståhl T, Lahtinen E (2006). *Towards closer intersectoral cooperation: the preparation of the Finnish national health report. Health in All Policies: prospects and potentials'*. Ståhl T, Wismar M, Ollia E, Lahtinen E, Leppo K. Helsinki, Ministry of Social Affairs and Health.

Ståhl T, Wismar M, et al. (2006). *Health in All Policies: prospects and potentials.* Helsinki, Finland.

Sukkumnoed D, Reukpornpipat K (2010). *Health impact assessment in Thailand: a learning tool for addressing Health in All Policies.* Implementing Health in All Policies: Adelaide 2010 Kickbusch I and Buckett K.

Vivian L, Jones C M, et al. (2012). *Synthesizing the evidence: how governance structures can trigger governance actions to support Health in All Policies. Intersectoral Governance for Health in All Policies Structures, actions and experiences.* McQueen D V, Matthias W, Vivian L, Jones C M, Davies M, World Health Organization on behalf of the European Observatory on Health Systems and Policies.

Whitehead M, Bird P (2008). *England. Health for all? A critical analysis of public health policies in eight European countries.* Hogstedt C, Moberg H, Lundgren B, Backhans M, Östersund Swedish National Institute of Public Health.

WHO working paper (2010). *School Health Promotion Program Case Study in Indonesia.*

WHO working paper (2010) *School Health Promotion Programme in Sri-Lanka*. Report prepared for WHO Sri Lanka.

WHO (2008a). *Social Determinants of Health.* Report of a Regional Consultation, Colombo, Sri Lanka, 2–4 October 2007.

WHO (2008b). *Country Cooperation Strategy at a Glance.* Accessed from http://www.who.int/countries/tha/en/

WHO (2009). *Programme on Reducing Harm from Alcohol Use in the Community.* Alcohol Control Series, Regional Office for South-East Asia. (No. 7).

WHO (2009). Regional Conference on Revitalizing Primary Health Care Jakarta, Indonesia, 6-8 August 2008 ".

WHO (2010a). *Follow-up action on pending issues and selected Regional Committee resolutions/decisions of the last three years: Nutrition and food safety in the South-East Asia Region* (SEA/RC60/R3) Regional Committee Provisional Agenda item 19.2, Sixty-third Session SEA/RC63/17. Bangkok, Thailand 7–10 September 2010 16 July 2010.

WHO (2010b). Policy Brief Scaling Up Nutrition: A Framework for Action. *Food and Nutrition Bulletin,* vol. 31(no. 1).

WHO (2011a). *Nutrition: Maternal, infant and young child nutrition: draft comprehensive implementation plan.* Report by the Secretariat Executive Board EB130/10, 130th session. Provisional agenda item 6.3.

WHO (2011b). *Intersectoral action on healthA path for policy-makers to implement effective and sustainable action on health*, WHO Centre for Health Development, Kobe.

WHO (2012a). *Background note: Meeting of Experts on Measuring Health Equity and Health Impact Assessment towards Health in all Policies,* WHO/SEARO, New Delhi. 6-8 June 2012. SEA/SDH-Meet.1/1 29 May 2012.

WHO (2012b). *Intersectoral actions for addressing social determinants of health.* Report of a regional consultation WHO-SEARO, New Delhi, 23-25 August 2011.

WHO (2012c). *Meeting Report: Bi-regional meeting on Scaling-up Nutrition, 10-12 August, 2011, Colombo, Sri Lanka.* World Health Organization Regional Office for South-East Asia, World Health Organization Regional Office for Western Pacific Department of Nutrition for Health & Development, WHO Geneva in collaboration with FAO, UNICEF, WFP and the World Bank.

WHO (2012d). *Non-communicable diseases including mental health and neurological disorders.* Report of the regional meeting, Yangon, Myanmar, 24–26 April 2012.

WHO (2012e). *Reducing Harm from Alcohol Use in the Community: Multiple Strategies Mental Health and Substance Abuse Unit,* Regional Office for South-East Asia, Reducing harm from alcohol use in the community: multiple strategies. (Alcohol Control Series No. 8)

WHO (2012f). *Regional consultation on safe street foods Bangkok, Thailand, 20–23 June, 2011 Bangkok, Thailand, 20–23 June, 2011,* Organized by World Health Organization Regional Office for South-East Asia Food and Agriculture Organization Regional Office for Asia and the Pacific Institute of Nutrition, Mahidol University, Thailand.

WHO (2012g). *Social Determinants of Health, Sri Lanka, Light-House Project.* World Health Organization, Sri Lanka.

WHO and Government of South Australia (2010). *Adelaide Statement on Health in All Policies, Adelaide.*

WHO and PHAC- Public Health Agency of Canada (2008). *Health Equity Through Intersectoral Action: An Analysis of 18 Country Case Studies.* Geneva: WHO.

WHO-Government of India Biennial work plan, 2012. *The role of intersectoral action in implementing the Framework Convention for Tobacco Control in India.* Final draft version (made available through WHO SEARO).